Life&Death

On The Streets

A **Paramedic's** Diary

Life&Death
On The Streets

STUART GRAY

LEARNING
RESOURCES
CENTRE

Monday Books

© **Stuart Gray 2007**
First published in Great Britain in 2007 by Monday Books

A CIP catalogue record for this title is available from
the British Library

2007 ISBN: 978-0-9552854-9-3

Printed and bound by Cox and Wyman
Typeset by Andrew Searle
Cover Design by Paul Hill at Kin Creative

www.mondaybooks.com
info@mondaybooks.com

Dedication

Dedicated to the memory of Tommy Gray, the man who encouraged me to believe in myself.

CONTENTS

Thanks

*My love and thanks to Jac, without you
I may not have stuck this out.
Thanks to Allan for holding the fort.
Thanks to all of my readers in the virtual world.
Thanks also to my friends and colleagues in the Service who
gave me encouragement and support, especially B, K, I and T.
Of course, my deepest thanks to the many hundreds of
patients who have become part of the diary and without
whom not a word of it would have been written.
Finally, thanks Scruffs...frequent interruptions for attention
helped break the monotony of writing!*

FOREWORD

This is an account of my working life as a paramedic in London. I came to the profession relatively late; I was a cub reporter back home in Scotland when I was only 16, spent a dozen years as a professional songwriter and musician, dabbled in business and computers through the late 80s and also did a three year stint with the Royal Army Medical Corps.

I finally settled on a pre-hospital career when I joined an ambulance service in Surrey. I underwent training to become a paramedic, in the days before the job title was protected as it is now, and when the training was a lot simpler. As the paramedical profession began to gain respect and importance in the ambulance service, I found myself out of the loop. I didn't work for the NHS and I couldn't continue using the title unless I became registered. So I completed a three year honours degree in Paramedic Science at the University of Hertfordshire (I got a first, which was an amazing personal achievement), got myself on the register and, well, the rest is history. (I nearly went for medicine but I missed UCAS registration by one month; it's still an option I might look at in the future).

Much of the material used in this book is drawn from my reflective diaries of the last four years. The more recent of these appear on my blog, 'The Paramedic's Diary' (you can read it at http://theparamedicsdiary.blogspot.com/ and you can email me from there if you like). It contains patient cases from my work as part of an ambulance crew and as a solo Fast Response Unit (FRU) paramedic, on my own in a car. When I describe situations where I'm with a crewmate, I'm in an ambulance, obviously. If I'm alone, I'm on the FRU.

Of course, some of it is skewed in favour of my own opinions and judgments but the call types, the emotions, the abuse and the hard work are all the same for everyone on the frontline.

Names, places and other details have been changed or omitted to preserve patient anonymity and confidentiality where consent has been impossible to obtain. This book is not endorsed in any way by the ambulance service I work for.

There are graphic details in some of the stories. Some of it will make you wince, but if I sanitised things it wouldn't reflect the job. There's not always a happy ending, and sometimes it's a heartbreaking job, but I do get to do some amazing things: my colleagues and I bring people back from the brink of death - I can't think of a better reason to write about my work than that.

HOAX CALLERS AND TIMEWASTERS

Regular callers are known as 'frequent flyers'.

Don't get me wrong, some people call us often because they need us often - they have genuine problems. But a few are just timewasters, draining the resources of the NHS by calling us just because they can.

They are dangerous people who cost lives, and there's not a damn thing we can do about it.

One old guy on my patch - I'm talking a man in his early 60s, at an age where he really should know better - calls 999 almost every other day. He has it down to a fine art: he knows when our shifts change and he times his call to coincide exactly with crew turnarounds, ensuring a speedy response and a fresh face or two. He rings for chest pain that he doesn't really have, abdominal problems that don't exist and various other complaints that he knows will guarantee him an emergency response. Partly, he likes the attention, partly he just likes to get a free ride down to the hospital where he's guaranteed more attention and a free lunch (or breakfast, or dinner). Some weeks, he'll have a car and an ambulance outside his home every day; if he visits a friend or goes off on holiday with family members, the calls stop - he never seems to get ill on those days.

I've 'treated' him many times, and on the last few occasions I've lectured him at length about what he is doing. He abuses his right to an ambulance over and over again, and yet nothing is done about it.

A while ago, he called us and I was despatched with my crewmate to his home. He was rude and arrogant, and he insisted on being carried down the stairs (there are no lifts where he lives, and he's on the third floor). He has no disability, and there was no medical reason that meant he needed to be carried, so we refused.

'Do you have any idea how many of us suffer with back pain because we have to carry people down stairs,' I said. 'I don't mind it when people can't walk or are seriously ill. But you can and you're not.'

He looked at me. 'But I've got chest pain,' he said. He knows full well we have to carry him if he's got 'chest pain', and so we did.

In the ambulance, I spoke to him once again about ringing 999 just so he can get to hospital and have his breakfast (he gets free sandwiches, and will call in the a.m. for breakfast or the p.m. for lunch). He ignored me, so I stopped talking and we sat in silence all the way to hospital.

We spent almost an hour with him, all told.

Halfway through, another call was broadcast over the radio. It was for an elderly lady 'trapped behind closed doors'. We could have been running to this call immediately, but we didn't get it until we 'greened up' after dropping our frequent flyer off at hospital.

GREENING UP: When a call is completed and the patient has been taken to hospital, we are required to 'green up'. This means hitting the 'green mobile' button on our systems so that EOC (control) can see that we are available for the next call. We also have a 'green at station' button so that they can call us at the station and 'green away from vehicle' so they can call us on a mobile phone when we're in the loo or buying a sarnie.

When we got to the trapped woman, she was dying behind her own front door. She had fallen the previous night and had been lying there ever since, her body preventing the door from opening so worried neighbours had been unable to get in to help her. We forced the door and I pushed my way into her hallway. She was now so weak that she could barely breathe. I gave her oxygen and we got her out as quickly as possible. It was an awkward, messy job, but we managed to get her to hospital within fifteen minutes of arriving.

But it was too late. She was pronounced dead soon afterwards.

We'd lost probably 45 minutes with our friend from earlier on. There's no way of knowing, but I believe that she would have had a chance if we'd got to her earlier. Even ten minutes might have made a difference, so it shouldn't surprise you that I blame that selfish, time-wasting old man for her death. It wasn't long before I was sent out to him again.

He was complaining of breathing difficulties which didn't exist.

'Last time you called me out,' I said, 'you delayed me getting to an old lady who had fallen and hurt herself.'

He looked at me, blankly.

'And you know what?' I said. 'She might not have died if you hadn't delayed us getting to her.'

He just sat there and shrugged his shoulders.

Other, less malicious people call us for what they perceive to be genuine emergencies but which turn out to be nothing of the sort.

I went to a one-month-old baby, *'? Suspended'* - the worst kind of call for me and no doubt for a lot of my colleagues. I really don't want to be holding someone's dead child and explaining to them that I had done the best I could, because that's a rubbish deal.

The call description stated 'not crying' and this was all the information I had when I set off. I called Control and asked them for a little bit more info. In fact, I asked them if I was going to a suspended baby or not. They replied that they were still taking the call so had nothing else to offer yet, except that they were treating this as a Red 1 - suspended.

When I arrived, an ambulance had just pulled up at the address and there was a motorcycle solo paramedic already inside. I felt that this must be a genuine dead baby - why else all the fuss? I went upstairs to the flat and entered the living room. I saw a very emotional mother, a worried relative, the ambulance crew, the solo paramedic and a baby lying on the floor. It was hiccupping.

The more liberal-natured among you may be persuaded that some of these people are simply 'uninitiated', or that their particular emergency is 'a true crisis for them'. Fine, but remember that *you* pay for this (annually, it's costing the tax-payer around £20m) and, more importantly, that one day it might be you or a loved one lying unable to breathe behind a door while we move someone's bed from one end of the room to the other because the *feng shui* isn't right, and the imbalance of *yin* and *yang* is giving them a headache.

It's not as though many people are unaware of the problem nowadays. The press often carry tales of the troublingly stupid calls that are received by the emergency services in this country. Here are a few recent ones:

A 31-year-old woman who dialled 999 because her TV remote control was out of reach.

Another 31-year-old who was worried because she had sniffed deodorant by accident.

A lazy father-to-be who demanded an ambulance for his wife; she was in labour but he couldn't take her to hospital himself because he was waiting for a pizza to be delivered.

A model who called Gloucestershire Ambulance Service when she broke her fingernail, for God's sake.

Some nutter who called the Scottish Ambulance Service to ask for a crew to come out and help wrap up Christmas presents.

My own ambulance service recently issued a press release pointing out that time-wasting calls were potentially costing lives; on the very day it was sent out, we took a call from a 22-

year-old woman who'd squeezed a spot which was now bleeding.

A pensioner told a frontline crew to wait 40 minutes before taking her to hospital because she was baking a cake. The crew gave her a warning and left - only for her to ring back exactly 40 minutes later.

Another phoned for an ambulance because her husband was refusing to listen to her. I wonder why?

The police get a lot of these dumb calls, too. Would you ring 999 to ask if your lost £20 note had been handed in, or to complain that your Chinese takeaway was cold? Or to try to sell the operator a pair of shoes? No. So who does? Ignorant timewasters.

NHS Direct have tried to help by supplying their website visitors with a list of situations which could be called true emergencies. These include unconsciousness, a suspected heart attack and suspected stroke. The trouble is that to a large section of the general public a sleeping drunk is 'unconscious', anyone with stomach ache or heartburn is suffering a suspected heart attack and many don't even understand what a stroke is, never mind diagnosing the possibility that one is occurring. (And on the subject of NHS Direct, calling them for advice is all well and good, but I've still been sent to calls where this has been done and the patient either hasn't been able to get through or has been told, unnecessarily, to call an ambulance anyway).

There's been talk of a new number, a sort of halfway house where you can call the emergency services but they won't have to rush out immediately - like they have in the United States, where you can dial 311 instead of 911 if your problem isn't too pressing. Unfortunately, the UK's telecoms industry regulator Ofcom dismissed the idea as impractical because of the massive and costly changes that it would have entailed. How typically British. Meanwhile, we still get called by people with shampoo in their eyes.

In my area, we do at least now have a screening system for not-really-emergency-calls. It's called Clinical Telephone Advice (CTA), and it's reasonably effective; trouble is, it can't weed out those who know how to play the system and who insist they have 'chest pain' or 'difficulty in breathing'.

* * * * *

Alongside the selfish and the stupid are the hoaxers. Across the country, almost 1,000 hoax calls are made to the ambulance service every week. Most are made by kids, bored out of their skulls and looking for stimulation and excitement; calling the emergency services ticks that box. You're almost certain not to get caught (though new technology is fast catching up) and you get to see blue flashing lights and hear sirens. As a special treat, you also get to see professional grown-ups scratching their heads and looking around aimlessly.

Some people just want to have a laugh at our expense. I was working on All Fool's Day when I received a call to a *'suicidal female - threatening to jump'*. I arrived with the police and we went to the location given, only to find that the place was a hostel and the staff knew nothing of a 999 call, let alone a potential suicide on the premises. We asked about the possibility of someone making the call from this place. We were told that there were no phones in the rooms, so we suggested that the payphone on the wall could have been used. That was impossible, they said, because nobody had been near it in the past few hours.

When the police got their Control to check the details again, they discovered that the call had originated *outside* of London. The hoax was confirmed when one of the hostel staff pointed out that, although we had a potentially suicidal female, this was an all-male hostel.

Sometimes hoax callers have an even more sinister agenda. A few years ago, a Bristol crew was pelted with stones by a gang of youths who had called 999 claiming a boy had fallen down stairs and then lay in wait for them at the scene. Others have been threatened with guns, knives and fists. Quite why anyone would want to do this is beyond me.

> **ABUSE. It's bizarre. We only exist to help people (and sometimes even save their lives). You'd think that everywhere we went there'd be grateful punters patting us on the back and doing whatever they could to help. Sometimes it is like that. Unfortunately, a lot of the time it's not. We get lots of abuse. All of it is supposed to be reported (there are forms to fill in) but since it ranges from something as minor as a swear word tossed in your direction to an outright physical attack, only the more significant events are ever reported. Otherwise, we would be filling in forms almost every shift and certainly every weekend. Nowadays, we wear ballistic stab vests, which says something. I'm told they will stop a .357 bullet, though I wouldn't like to prove it. But they will stop knives and you hardly feel punches and kicks. We get punched and kicked a lot. During the summer season, when everyone gets tanked up outside, and over Christmas, it happens every week. It's almost always drunks.**

We all get these 'unknown caller, unknown problem, please investigate' calls; most are thoroughly mundane and only a few of those I've received are worth talking about. Most of them result in a short area search, a bit more paperwork than is necessary and a frustrated paramedic or ambulance crew. Of course, some of them cost lives. The odd one shows a bit more thought and deserves a mention for the sheer audacity of the perpetrators (though that doesn't mean they don't deserve locking up for a month or so).

A few years ago, when I was working at another station, we were called to a 'dead child in the street'. It was about ten o'clock at night and quite dark when we arrived at the small residential estate. There were two young police officers standing over what looked like the lifeless body of a young child. It was dressed in a tracksuit and a bright red jacket, and was lying face down in the gutter. There was a pool of blood around the head.

My crewmate, who was attending, got out of the vehicle and went over to check it out. I followed behind and saw that she was about to try for a response from the person on the ground. Then she gave it a funny look and grabbed the head, pulling it up and forward to reveal the 'child' underneath.

It was a dummy.

The kids on the street, no doubt watching from the shadows, had created a beautifully realistic corpse, with a face drawn on a cardboard 'head' attached to a teddy bear's torso. The legs and arms of the tracksuit had been stuffed with socks to give it a realistically human shape, and it was wearing a pair of Nike Airs. It was very effective, especially in the half-light of the street lamps.

The blood, as I discovered when I touched it with my gloved hand, was tomato ketchup.

The kids had dumped it on the pavement and then called the cops. The two officers had shown up but hadn't even bothered to touch it to investigate (they were wary and wanted us to do that for them). Unfortunately, when my crewmate showed them what it was they had to admit that they'd already called CID and were waiting for them to arrive. I've never seen redder-faced police officers, and I always wondered what the Detective Inspector said to them when he got there.

We took the offending article back to our ambulance station and hung it up on the wall as a reminder. Over the next few weeks it slowly disappeared as parts of it (the clothing was new and of good quality) were taken away by crews.

Not all timewasting calls are made on purpose. One little girl phoned 999 to complain that her mum had forgotten to feed the cat. You'd have to have a heart of stone not to laugh at that.

SEEING DEAD PEOPLE

Some patients are more memorable than others, regardless of age or background.

I remember one lady very clearly: she was a lovely little Greek granny in her 70s. I met her at St Bart's Hospital - she had cancer and she needed conveying elsewhere for an MRI scan. As I attended her, we chatted and laughed; we just got on very well and it was almost like I was her long-lost grandson or something. I'd meet her from time to time, when I was doing patient transfers, and she always had a big grin and a wisecrack or two.

I mention her because I'd seen her at St Bart's one afternoon, and that night my then boss said he wanted to take me down to the morgue. I hadn't been exposed to death, and he thought it would be a good idea for me to go and sit in there and look at dead people. It sounds morbid, and no-one relishes it, but death is an occupational hazard and your first corpse is one of the things you most want to get out of the way when you start working in pre-hospital care.

Still, I was nervous, obviously, and I had this strange fear that I'd see someone who was dead wake up. Anyway, I knew it had to be done and I wanted to get it over with. We walked past a number of shrouded figures, and then he said, 'Do you remember this person?'

He had a big grin on his face as he pulled back the sheet. It was my old Greek lady, lying there, eyes closed, looking for all the world as though she was just asleep. I had seen her three or four hours earlier, full of life, and we'd had a good chat. No hint that she was going to die. Now here she was. It was a kick in the teeth, and I still think it was the cruellest thing ever done to me, considering how well I had been getting on with her and how suddenly she had gone.

'ATTENDING'. With ambulance calls, one person drives and the other 'attends' the patient, and actually treats them; the following day, you swap roles.

After that, trips to the local hospital to watch post mortems became a regular event for me and some of my colleagues. Not only did my fear of seeing dead people eventually evaporate, but my knowledge of real anatomy increased. It's a mile off from talking about the human heart and how a heart attack affects it to actually seeing one being removed from a person's chest, hours after they have died, and looking at the scarred evidence of a myocardial infarction.

MYOCARDIAL INFARCTION, or 'MI', means heart attack. It describes the death of the heart muscle (not all of it, but a part of it) due to lack of oxygen as a result of ischaemia (lack of blood flow, meaning little or no oxygen is being delivered). The word 'infarction' comes from the Latin 'infarcire', meaning 'to plug up or cram', and it refers to the clogging of the artery that results in a lack of oxygen to part of the heart muscle (the myocardium). Myocardial means 'of the heart muscle'.

Interestingly, the only pink lungs you ever see belong to relatively young people. Smokers or not, the lungs of all the adults I've seen being dissected are blackened and sooty from the everyday pollution we live with. The pathologists will tell you they rarely see good quality lungs, even from those living in the countryside.

Over the years (and that first exposure to death was more than 15 years ago now), I've become accustomed to seeing corpses in various stages of decomposition. The dead don't unnerve me, but the surprise of finding them does. Even today, a call to a 'person trapped behind locked doors' with a history of not having been seen for days (or even weeks) can give me the creeps. I know I'll have to go into the house and that I'll probably find them dead somewhere. There'll be a terrible smell and the place will be buzzing with bluebottles. Every room becomes a horrible adventure.

I went to a call like this with a colleague a few weeks ago. The woman hadn't been seen or heard of for a few days and we had reason to believe that she might need urgent emergency help, so we decided to kick the door in. (We asked her relatives for permission; they were standing anxiously by, as was a gaggle of curious neighbours and her local church minister, who was worried about her lack of attendance at the recent Sunday service.)

My colleague gave the door a couple of hefty kicks, in it went and so did we. We looked in every room and eventually found her in the bath - dead. A little trickle of blood had escaped her mouth and her head hung across her shoulder as if she'd fallen asleep. There was no water in the bath; it had either slowly leaked out through the plug or had never been put in, but that didn't matter to her now. The police arrived shortly afterwards to take over the scene, checking for evidence of foul play or forced entry. The front door was the only thing that showed entry by force and we were the culprits.

The grief of relatives can be overwhelming to witness. More often than not there's a quiet, muffled sobbing going on in one of the other rooms as you inspect a corpse for confirmation. Sometimes you get a lot more emotion than that.

I was with a crewmate on a long and very busy night shift a while back when we were called to a 'suspended' - as in between life and death, not breathing, no pulse, in cardiac arrest. 'Suspended' means someone thinks there's a chance we might be able to save the patient by starting CPR when we get on scene. Unfortunately, this is sometimes down to wishful thinking, as it was in this case. The man was on the floor of his bedroom and had been dead for at least an hour.

> CPR stands for cardiopulmonary resuscitation, an emergency medical procedure for victims of cardiac or respiratory arrest. Blood circulation and breathing are stimulated artificially by chest compression and lung ventilation. The idea is to try to maintain a flow of oxygenated blood to the brain and the heart, delaying tissue death and extending the window of opportunity for successful resuscitation using defibrillation and life support systems.

He'd rolled in after a night of drinking with his best friend and lodger, a young, red-haired man whose face I will never forget. He'd sat up with his wife and the red-haired man until about 2am, then, feeling a little worse for wear, had gone to have a lie down in bed. Some time had passed and the wife had got fed up shouting for him to come and get something to eat. She'd gone up into the bedroom and found him lying very still in bed. Either she couldn't work out what was going on, or she'd gone into immediate denial, but she'd asked the red-haired man to check him. He did and fled the room to call an ambulance when he realised his mate wasn't breathing.

Following instructions given over the phone by the call-taker, he had dragged the man off the bed and tried to carry out CPR but was woefully unable to do it because he didn't fully understand the instructions and his emotions weren't under control.

When we arrived, he virtually pulled us into the bedroom and then left to comfort his mate's wife - widow, now - in the front room downstairs. She didn't want to come near us in case we told her something she didn't want to hear... I understood that fear. We checked the man's vitals and found that he had none: he had been on the floor for some time and was purple plus. He had a long history of liver disease and a dubious cardiac health record and, anyway, he was already stiff at the fingers and around the face. CPR would be useless. The decision was made not to attempt resuscitation.

We went into the front room and found the young man sitting in tears on a chair. The new widow was pacing the room and looked out of her head. We broke the bad news to them as quickly and softly as humanly possible.

'There's nothing we can do for him, I'm afraid,' my colleague said.

That single sentence provoked a long and anguished wail from the woman and a sudden emotional collapse in the red-haired man. We had to stay with them for quite a while; we'd requested police, which is normal procedure in these cases, but they were delayed and couldn't guarantee being with us for several hours. During that long wait with the two closest people in the dead man's life, the other guy's eyes never dried. He looked like a scared puppy and he kept repeating the same thing over and over again: 'What am I going to do now?'

Apparently, the older man was his only friend and he had nowhere to live but this house. The woman seemed to shun him and I got the impression she somehow blamed him for her husband's death. When she eventually calmed down, she left the room after asking if she could see her husband again. I went with her; she kissed him on the forehead and lips. It was agonising to watch. Real grief reminds you of your own loved ones and I kept thinking about how horrible this will feel when it happens to me, as it inevitably will.

I left her alone with him for a few minutes while she said her final goodbyes. Then she came back into the front room and never spoke to any of us again after that.

The cops arrived soon afterwards, and that started a fresh torrent of despair. We left, the police officers not knowing where to look or what to do.

* * * * *

I travelled a long way into south London for another 'suspended', but, again, there was no work to be done. An ambulance was already on scene when I pulled up outside the small terraced house. The front door was wide open and people were milling around in the hallway. One of the crew came to meet me and just shook her head. I went upstairs to see what I could do, if anything, but the man was dead in his bed, and had been for a while. He was stone cold and rigor mortis was just creeping in to his peripheries.

The man's wife was in the room, along with her daughters and a son.

'His eyes are still open,' she said to me

'Do you want me to close them?' I asked.

'But his eyes are open,' she repeated.

I went over to the bed and together we closed his eyes for the last time.

Then she said the same thing that many others have said in this situation. 'What am I going to do now?'

And she began to cry. I put an arm around her shoulder until a relative took over. I left the house and the crew stayed behind to complete their paperwork and manage the family's grief until the doctor or police arrived.

'PURPLE'. We call the recently dead 'purple' and those who have been dead a while 'purple-plus'. The morgue is referred to as the 'purple annexe'.

Last month I answered a call for a 'female, possibly trapped behind a locked door'. I raced round to the address and the police got there a few moments later. It turned out the 'woman' was actually a male called Dave and his brother Andy was waiting there anxiously for us to arrive. He'd knocked - and then hammered - on the door to the flat and got no response, so he'd then visited his brother's few regular haunts and found no sign there either. Dave hadn't been seen for three days now, so Andy had rung 999.

I looked through the letterbox and sniffed the air inside: there was no unusual smell, but a light was on in the front room. I shouted through but there was no reply, just a dead quiet. The door was very well secured and the police officer had no luck trying to kick it in. One of them went to fetch the 'key' - a battering ram used to smash down doors - but while he was gone the brother unscrewed a piece of plywood covering a small, broken window. The other police officer, who was a slip of a girl, was able to squeeze herself in through the gap and open the door from the inside. I made my way in, and the brother followed. He noticed that Dave's inhalers were still on the table, along with other personal effects that would normally be with him if he went out, so that didn't look great. We went from room to room, me expecting to find a corpse in any one of them. We'd checked the living room, the kitchen and the bedroom, and the brother started to relax. 'Thank God,' he said, with evident relief. 'He must be out somewhere.'

But he spoke too soon. We were all heading out of the flat through the small hallway when I noticed the bathroom door ajar. I'd assumed it had been cleared, but I looked through the gap between the door and the wall anyway. Dave was inside, sitting on the loo. I signalled to the police officer that I'd found him and that his brother should be kept back for a moment. I went in and checked him. He was pulseless, cold and stiff.

Andy pushed past me and fell apart. He cried all the way out of the flat. I felt sorry for him, but I couldn't help him and I had nothing to offer. He called his wife and told her what had happened, sobbing through the entire call, trying and failing to keep his composure. He was still in tears when I left.

You try to be as respectful as possible, obviously. Occasionally, something embarrasses you. I was called to confirm life extinct on a male who had been found by his regular carer and neighbour. The guy was sitting in a chair in front of the telly, a half-opened nebuliser in his hands and cans of beer strewn around the floor - one of which was waiting to be opened.

The carer had let himself in to give the man some breakfast, only to find him sitting upright, for all the world looking as though he was watching the birds in his garden. He was asthmatic and had emphysema, and had a home oxygen system and a portable, mains-powered nebuliser compressor. It looked as if he had suffered an attack and had attempted to give himself some salbutamol but that at the crucial moment his electricity meter had run out of credit and the power had failed. The compressor stopped working and he had gone, very quickly, in the middle of trying to save himself.

As I sat there, my service mobile phone rang. Some joker had reset the ring-tone to the sound of a rooster.

> **EMTs are Emergency Medical Technicians. They are highly-trained and skilled and make up most of the population of the ambulance service, but they are not paramedics; paramedics have more advanced skills and are qualified to use invasive techniques and drugs which EMTs are not. All paramedics were once EMTs and many EMTs will go onto become paramedics.**

It doesn't always end in tears. Last year I went to a house where the tenant hadn't been seen for 24 hours and his dog - which was large and known to be highly protective - was barking relentlessly inside. The police were there and an officer with a mirror on a stick had cautiously crept up the stairs and located the animal with the makeshift periscope. It was on the bed, staring angrily right at him, and it had bounded off, growling, sending him scuttling back downstairs. He'd seen no body, but it seemed a fair bet that the owner was probably unconscious or dead on the bedroom floor. If that was the case, the canine protector wasn't going to let anyone near him; we could all hear it panting and growling to itself at the top of the stairs. Nervously, I checked the fit of my stab vest and then thought, *'Who am I kidding?'*

So I stood at the bottom of the stairs with two coppers and the neighbour who'd called us. No ambulance was yet free and the dog handler was a good 30 minutes away.

As we waited, we discussed the tenant's habits and medical conditions with the neighbour, trying to build up a picture of what might have happened to him. He had a long history of heart problems and he never, ever left the house without his dog, she said. The back door had been left unlocked. Things were looking dire.

After a while, and with still no sight of the dog handler, I decided to use the mirror to have another go at establishing if there was a body in the room.

The first thing I saw (and I can tell you my breathing rate was a lot faster than normal) was a huge Alsatian on the bed. He was looking straight into the mirror at me, with angry eyes and a mouth-full of nasty-looking teeth. I didn't have much of a horizon to view, and I couldn't see the man. But he could easily have been elsewhere. It did occur to me that the dog might have eaten him - stranger things have happened - but I dismissed the thought and put it down to nerves.

I craned my neck, trying to see further into the bedroom. Every second or two, my eyes flicked back to the dog; my horror-movie fear was that I'd be scanning the floor as he crept nearer to me, fangs bared. All I'd see were two rows of teeth and a dribble of saliva, followed by a messy end (mine, not his). I still saw nothing of his master.

I came back down the stairs and waited with the other nervous people below. The dog was still snarling and growling menacingly upstairs. Suddenly, and very nonchalantly, a man opened the back door and strode in. A look of shock flashed across his face at the sight of two policemen and a paramedic standing in his hallway. Then he recovered himself.

'Can I help you at all?' he asked.

'Are you the tenant of this property, sir?' said one of the police officers.

'Yes, what's going on - why are you all here?'

Meanwhile, the neighbour is trying to curl up into the smallest ball in the known universe.

'We were called because your dog was howling and barking and the neighbour thought you were in trouble,' said the cop.

'I'm OK. I just went out for the night to visit my sister.'

'Do you always go out without locking your doors, sir?'

'Yes.'

I could hear the siren of the police dog van approaching. The dog handler would get out of his vehicle, get his equipment prepared and be told to stand down. He would be so disappointed. I had to smile.

The man went up to see his dog and brought it down to say hello to us. Everyone took a step or two back, but it just walked by, wagging its tail and licking the owner's hand, and didn't even look at us.

TRAFFIC

It's getting worse everywhere, isn't it? In London, it's beyond bad these days. Despite the higher charges and ludicrous taxes, despite the congestion charging and speed camera rip-offs, our traffic problems are greater now than ever before. Expensive and unreliable public transport systems don't encourage people out of their cars, and driving to work is still often cheaper and easier than travelling by any other method.

For a paramedic, this increase in traffic means more accidents than ever. Though we're supposed to call them 'collisions' now.

Despite that, the chances of you dying in an RTC are still low, and the number of road deaths has remained fairly constant over the last ten years. Around half of those who do wind up dead on the road are car drivers, around a fifth are on motorbikes and the rest are spread around cyclists, bus drivers and hauliers. Oh, and pedestrians.

> **RTC. Road Traffic Collision. We used to say RTA (Road Traffic Accident) but someone, somewhere, decided the word 'accident' meant that nobody was to blame and potentially posed a legal nightmare. Now, no matter what hits what (eg bike vs. pedestrian, bus vs. car, cyclist vs. manhole cover), someone can be held accountable, although I'd like to see what a manhole cover has to say for itself in court.**

Early one cold, foggy Friday morning last December, I was sent to a fatal RTC, called in by an off-duty policeman who'd seen a car swerve in front of him and had then seen a body lying in the road.

Traffic

It had happened outside a tube station; I raced there hoping, as I always do, that there'd been a mistake and the word 'fatal' had been used by accident.

When I arrived there was a queue of traffic blocking my way and vehicles were being reversed out. There was a flurry of activity up ahead and I could see flashing blue lights. I drove down the wrong side of the road to get to the scene and an ambulance followed behind me.

I swung my car around - I was on the FRU at the time - and my headlights lit up a body in the middle of the road, completely uncovered and obviously dead. It was a man and half his head had disappeared. I got out of the car and walked over.

The nearby pubs and clubs were chucking out and loose groups of people were standing around the railings at the side of the pavement; knots of young men and women staring at the mangled body a few yards away. Some, shockingly, disgustingly, were taking photos with their mobile phones.

I crouched down and examined his injuries. He was in his twenties, dressed for a night out drinking and clubbing. His skull had been crushed, leaving a large pool of blood on the road, and his intestines had burst from his abdomen and were lying on the road just in front of him. He wasn't long dead: an eerie plume of steam was rising into the cold air from his exposed organs. His limbs were all horribly out of shape and place.

I went back to the car and got a blanket. I had used it half an hour earlier to keep a drunken 18-year-old warm; now it was going to cover this young man's body before anyone else decided to take pictures of it. Although there were lots of people knocking around, no-one seemed to know what had happened to him - even his mate, who was now with the police, had no idea how he'd come to be lying dead in the middle of the road.

As I covered the body up, I noticed there was a club's wrist tag lying nearby. His trainers had been forced off his feet and were lying at different locations near his body; body parts, which had been forced out by whatever had hit him (and it must have been something big and heavy), were on the Tarmac. I got some yellow clinical waste bags and covered everything on the road that had belonged to him or been him.

Another ambulance had now arrived. Sadly, there was nothing we could do, but we couldn't move the body, either: this was a crime scene and we had to wait for forensics. So I sat near the body, in the damp, early morning air, listening to the sounds of London around me, pondering. It looked like a straightforward hit-and-run, where the guy had left a club and simply been run over as he walked across the road. But the more I thought about it, the less likely that seemed. His position and injuries didn't equate to a straightforward stand-up collision with a couple of tons of vehicle. No, he'd been lying down when he'd been struck. I think he'd climbed the pavement barrier and lain down in the middle of the road to sleep. He was probably very drunk, and, for some reason, drunks sometimes do this. I think he was right there, on this busy road, covered in a shroud of rolling fog, when a vehicle came round the corner and ran over him. He was a small man and his clothing was dark; it wouldn't have been easy to see him. The vehicle had destroyed his head and mid-torso instantly, rolling the body a few times. The driver had then carried on, either because he hadn't realised what he'd just done - I've heard of a similar incident, where the driver thought he'd gone over a bin bag when he'd actually just killed someone - or because he was so shocked and terrified that he didn't know what else to do. Alternatively - and this is a possibility, these days - he just didn't care.

Whatever happened, it was all over very quickly. It makes you think: the lad had probably had a shower, splashed on his favourite after-shave, got dressed up and gone out. On any other night, he might have met the woman he'd marry, or had a kebab and gone home. But on this night, when he'd shut his front door, he had six hours to live.

Some RTCs involve horrific injuries that are still survivable if the right action is taken. Rapid Sequence Induction (RSI) is carried out in emergencies where there is a need to quickly intubate a patient in order to preserve the airway and lungs. I took a night-time call to a 'Car vs. Pedestrian' in a distant part of town. I didn't think I'd get to it - it was in an area that I normally get cancelled down on before I arrive. In fact, when I got on scene there was a crew already in attendance - a paramedic and an EMT. They were working around a large male who looked either unconscious or dead in the road. The paramedic broke away for a second or two to tell me that the guy had been unconscious since being hit by a car at an unknown speed a few minutes earlier. A Delta Alpha - our term for a rapid response doctor - had been called.

RSI involves putting the patient to sleep using an anaesthetic; this relaxes the muscles so that they cannot breathe for themselves and have no gag reflex, so we then intubate them. This means inserting an endotracheal (ET) tube into the trachea (windpipe); this is sealed so that only the air being pushed through it will enter the lungs. Fluids and other obstructions from the mouth and the contents of the stomach will not be able to get down the trachea - this guarantees a secure airway for the patient. The tube feeds into a cylindrical plastic bag, which is in turn fed by an oxygen bottle. We squeeze this cylinder in a rhythm which mimics breathing, forcing oxygen down the tube and into the lungs, artificially inflating them and oxygenating the blood. Only Delta Alphas - emergency doctors - can perform RSI, and, in the ambulance service, only paramedics can intubate.

I crouched down alongside my colleagues. I could see that the man had sustained a serious head injury but we could find no other significant or obvious trauma to the rest of his body. His neck was stabilised and an oropharyngeal airway (OP) had been inserted to keep his tongue from obstructing his airway. He was breathing and he had a strong pulse, but when I lifted his eyelids to check his pupils his eyeballs were rolling from side to side, a sign of possible brain injury. He also had blood coming from his left ear, so a basal skull fracture was likely. The guy was in serious trouble.

We got him into the ambulance and began to gather all the information we needed for our baseline obs. His breathing was unpredictable (shallow, then deep), and he needed assistance with a bag-valve-mask while I got on with cannulating him so I could run fluids through his veins if necessary.

CANNULATION. A cannula is a plastic tube designed for insertion into a body cavity. We use a cannula for the nasal-delivery of oxygen, and paramedics also use venous cannulae, incorporating a sheathed needle which is inserted into a vein (cannulation) so that fluids and drugs may be delivered. Paramedics will decide on an appropriate size (IV cannula sizing is all about bore width - how wide the hollow part of the needle is) depending on: the age and size of the patient, the size and condition of their veins and the amount of fluid or drugs that are to be given. Larger bore cannulae are chosen for trauma and cardiac arrest, simply because fluids will almost always be given. It is common for paramedics to choose a middle-sized cannula (18g) for most patients requiring IV access because this will enable a choice of drugs and fluids if required. Paramedics may also decide to cannulate a patient so that a vein is made 'patent', in case his condition deteriorates and finding an appropriate vein becomes difficult later on. This technique is known as 'Keep Vein Open' (KVO).

The Delta Alpha arrived. As he did so, the man began to stir, probably awoken by the oxygen. The doctor quickly RSI-d him, feeding a sedative in through the tubes I'd inserted.

As the drug went in, the man started thrashing around. We call this being 'combative'. People with massive head injuries can become very combative, and it's amazing and frightening to see. Essentially, the higher brain has 'shut down' and the person is operating at an instinctive level, with the pre-modern brain stem in charge - it summons up huge amounts of adrenaline, which in turn summons up a huge amount of strength. (It's for this reason that soldiers in battle report that they are unaware of physical exertion, and how terrified people manage to perform amazing feats of strength - a mother lifting a car off her child, for instance.) Injured people can become almost superhuman and it can take three or four of you just to hold them down; I have seen people hurled - in fact, *I've* been hurled - around ambulances by tiny folks who you wouldn't look twice at. Obviously, this is dangerous: as they flail about they can easily injure themselves - or us - and break equipment. Blood and tissue is flying around.

Luckily, in this case, almost as soon as he became combative he was out again, thanks to the RSI. He was already bagged, and now we gave him fluids to replace his lost blood; his condition stabilised and he was ready to go to hospital.

I got in my car and led the ambulance there as rapidly as possible, using my vehicle to clear a path, helping to ensure a smooth ride for the patient and those in the back with him.

We got him into Resus and he was quickly taken for a CT scan. His chances of survival should be good, but if the initial crew on scene, or me, had been delayed by a matter of minutes - maybe by one of those hoax callers - he'd have been dead or very seriously impaired. He was a married man with a couple of young kids; we did a good job that day.

OBS. Short for 'observations'. Initial clinical obs are carried out for every patient, and they include the vital signs; respiration rate, pulse rate, blood pressure and temperature. Other clinical obs include oxygen saturation level, capillary refill duration, BM (blood glucose) measurement, pupil responses and possibly an ECG (an electrocardiogram measures electrical activity in the heart). Generally speaking, an EMT or paramedic will decide which of the non-vital signs require further investigation, although our guidelines direct us to carry out many of them routinely. Two full sets of obs are required if a patient is to be left at home or in the care of another person.

Of course, as you stand over a bleeding, semi-conscious bloke lying in the middle of the road, you can't concern yourself with his family. You have to keep your emotions in check, however hard that can be. I went to another RTC where a group of teenagers crammed into a small car had sped down a hill and smashed straight into a big, brick wall. No brakes had been applied - there were no skid marks - and they must have hit it at 50 or 60mph. The wall hadn't yielded, so the car and the people inside had taken most of the force from the impact.

The scene was one of devastation and the LFB (London Fire Brigade - they cut people out of cars for us, hold up fluid bags and give everyone oxygen, and they also rescue cats and do stuff with fires) were already on scene with another ambulance when I arrived. Two of the four youngsters in the vehicle had already been taken to hospital with serious injuries, another was in the ambulance that had arrived ahead of us and we were to extricate and convey the last casualty - a young girl of fifteen who was trapped inside on the passenger's side.

It took us more than 15 minutes to get her out of the car. She screamed and cried throughout the entire process, and thrashed around, making it impossible to give her morphine. She was yelling about the pain in her legs, and it was thought she may have broken both femurs. This was a life-threatening injury.

We get her out, a pretty young kid with her whole life in front of her, and into the ambulance as quick as we can. Hold her down. Talk to her. She's not listening. In fact, she's wailing and kicking those broken legs about. The restraints can hardly hold her. She's in agony. Her pelvis may be broken, too. Not a moment too soon, the Delta Alpha arrives. She is RSI-d.

So now she's asleep, which is good, but we have to keep her alive. This is an awesome responsibility.

She was breathing on her own 60 seconds ago. Albeit in a lot of pain, but she was breathing. Now I'm breathing for her, with the bag.

If she dies, it will be my fault. No-one else to blame.

Intubating sounds easy - stick a tube down the throat, how hard can that be? Well, imagine it's dark, you've got seconds to work with, there might be blood in the mouth… if I don't get the tube directly into her lungs, via her trachea, the chances are that 80% of this air will instead go directly into her stomach. If it goes into her stomach, it's not going into her lungs. It will also inflate her stomach, which will cause her to vomit. And then she'll be screwed, because her already starved airway is now blocked with puke. Vomit is the biggest complication in resuscitation and can indirectly kill people.

I get the tube in correctly, and she doesn't vomit.

We blue her in and I bag her until she arrives at hospital, where the trauma team take over her life support and work out their treatment strategy.

Her weeping parents arrive and stand at her side as the medics begin their work. Quite distressing, the whole thing, and you can't help putting your own kids in that position and seeing yourself in the parents' place.

I learned a few months later that she had survived - it was touch and go - and was well on her way to recovery. She remembered nothing of the accident, or of the chaos that had ensued.

> **BLUED-IN. Taken to hospital on blue lights and sirens. Time-critical and life-threatening injuries and illnesses are conveyed like this. It's a clinical judgment call sometimes and it can be embarrassing if it's incorrectly judged. EOC - our Emergency Operations Centre, from where every ambulance in London is monitored, directed and supported - will call the receiving hospital on their 'red phone' and the Resus department will be made ready for the patient (and lots of medical students will turn up out of thin air).**

One of my recent RTC calls involved two cars, a bus and an unknown number of casualties. I'd just completed a long and very busy 12-hour shift. I should have been heading for home but this call had come in at the last minute. Driving on blue lights when you are tired is a surreal experience, but training, experience and caution keep you safe and the co-operation of the other drivers on the road - when you get it - helps a lot, too.

It was the beginning of the week, and the rush to get to work had begun in earnest.

I arrived just ahead of my colleagues. A bus was parked at an odd angle on this very busy main road, and a van was across the way from it. Opposite that was a badly mangled Vauxhall - it turned out to be a minicab - sitting in the middle of the road with a gaggle of police officers and fire-fighters peering in. The driver and his heavily-bloodied woman passenger were trapped inside - the impact had squashed the roof down somehow, and smashed the doors in and up so that they couldn't be opened. An FRU colleague was leaning in through the side window, controlling the passenger's head and neck. She had a severe head injury, but was conscious and seemed alert and strangely calm. The driver was sitting quietly, not moving a muscle, staring out of his windscreen at the commotion that was unfolding around him. It's weird how people react in situations like this: some become hysterical, others seem content to trust you to get them out OK.

The best thing I could do was to help the man. I grabbed a fire-fighter and asked him to smash the rear windscreen for me, which he did. Wiping as much of the broken glass away as I could, I climbed into the car and slid myself in down next to the woman. She couldn't see properly for the blood in her eyes, but she must have felt or heard me because she reached out and groped around on the seat until she found my left hand. Then she grabbed it just about as tight as it's ever been grabbed. And she absolutely would not let go.

I could smell petrol, but LFB were already spreading sand on the road. They're hot on this, unsurprisingly. I looked around the driver and saw that the ignition was still on. 'Guys,' I shouted, 'can someone pop the bonnet and disconnect the battery.' No-one wants to be stuck in a car wreck with sparks and fuel flying around.

With my free hand, I tried to hold the driver's head still so a collar could be put on him to protect his cervical spine. Anyone involved in any high velocity RTC will be put in a collar.

And there I sat. The woman, not looking at me, said, 'Can you call my husband please? Could somebody call my husband?'

A fire-fighter said he would, but he must have forgotten; she kept worrying on about the call, and I could understand why. She was frightened, she'd been in a nasty accident and she was trapped in a car and surrounded by strangers. She asked again, 'Has anyone called my husband?'

I leaned forward and yelled, 'Look, could somebody please call her husband? Get the number and call him.'

29

And a young fireman came over and made the call. To me, putting her mind at rest was almost as important as dealing with her medical issues.

The driver was complaining of numbness in his neck but by now another crew had got his collar on and he was being given oxygen.

The LFB brought over their cutting gear and started taking the roof off. I seemed to sit there inside that wrecked Vauxhall for an age, with the fire crew sawing and tugging at the metal. The noise and smoke it makes can be very disturbing, especially if you've just been in a car crash; the woman was now crushing my hand. As soon as the roof was clear, she was lifted out and taken away very quickly. Because the driver had possible neck and spine injuries, we couldn't scoop him out; he had to sit a while longer while the firefighters cut his door away.

Once we got him to the ambulance it began to look as though he'd been very lucky and had suffered no more than a cut to his head. But the crash had been so powerful that we couldn't rule out more serious injury, so he was taken into Resus where his passenger was already being treated.

We have three CALL CATEGORIES, which are the Government's way of ensuring you get the best service from us (when actually more funds and more staff are what we really need). They are A, B and C, otherwise known as Red, Amber and Green. Category A/Red calls - get there very fast. (Dead, suspended, in serious trouble. Drunk and knows how to work the system.) Category B/Amber calls - get there fast. (Pregnant. Was ill but feeling better. Drunk and not sure how to work the system.) Category C/Green calls - get there at some point in the day. (Minor injury, certainly not life threatening. Lonely. Drunk and honest.)

I got chatting to a couple of the police who were there; they'd been sitting at traffic lights when they noticed the bus heading straight for a red light. They'd stuck on their blue lights to warn him but he'd continued and rammed straight into the taxi, which had spun and hit the van behind it. There was a large 'bull's-eye' on the car's windscreen; it took me ages to figure out that it had been caused by the driver's mobile phone flying out of its holder as the bus hit it.

Funnily enough, on my way back from this job a taxi came careering out of a side street and nearly T-boned me.

Not everyone is killed *by* a car. Some people just die *in* them.

The Man Who Went Shopping And Never Came Home is one of the strangest vehicle calls I've attended. He was a 59-year-old chap who had nipped out to the shops at around 8am and just disappeared. His family reported him missing in mid-afternoon. The police were out looking for him, but it was his son who made the discovery. He'd been called by his mum at lunchtime and asked to come home from work because she couldn't find his dad anywhere. He was scouring the local residential streets, using the roads that he knew his dad would have used to get to and from the shops, when he found him, dead in his car.

By the time we arrived, the police were already on scene and the son was in the background talking to them.

I approached the car and there was a middle-aged fellow inside, sitting at the wheel as if he was ready to go at any second. The key was in the ignition, his hands were rested on his lap and his head was bowed. He didn't look as if he had suffered at all. There was a small pool of vomit on the road on the driver's side. He must have pulled over feeling ill, opened the door, vomited, closed the door again and promptly died of a massive heart attack.

And there he'd sat, all morning and well into the afternoon, while the kids played outside and the mums walked up and down pushing buggies, and nobody, not a single person, took any notice of him.

Now he was the centre of attention, though, as we gathered around the car to plan his removal. The neighbours were twitching their curtains and standing in small, hushed groups, some saying they'd known something wasn't quite right with him, others that they'd thought he was just sleeping (without moving, all day).

It took us some time to get him out of the vehicle because he was tall and now he was also stiff. In the end, we had to put him on a spinal board and take him out as if he was a live RTC casualty. He wasn't, of course; he was someone's dad and someone's husband and he just didn't make it home.

STRONG ARM TACTICS

Fractures are common and you'll treat loads if you join the ambulance service. Lots happen in RTCs or other accidents, but some are a bit more bizarre in origin. Take arm-wrestling, for instance.

The first time I encountered this type of injury, I couldn't believe what I was hearing. We'd been called to a flat in the early hours of a Sunday morning for a young guy who'd 'damaged his arm'. The call was vague, at best, and my colleague and I expected to find the victim of an assault, or someone who'd been drunk and had fallen over.

We go to the address and went upstairs to the front room. We found a teenager sitting on a wooden chair with his smirking mates standing around him. He was holding his right arm gingerly and wincing in pain whenever he moved.

I asked what had happened and there was a murmuring from the small group around him. He looked sheepish. Then he piped up. 'I was arm wrestling my mate,' he said. 'I think it's broken.'

I raised my eyebrows - *Yeah, right* - and looked around the room. All I could see were stupid grins and empty beer cans. Stella, mostly. Maybe he was telling the truth. I knew about spiral fractures, where a break can occur as a result of wrenching or twisting forces, but *arm wrestling*? Come on. Turns out it's actually surprisingly easy to do, especially with enough booze inside you. Drunken arm-wrestlers have 'reduced proprioception' - in layman's terms, they're off their faces, so they forget to stop wrestling when it starts hurting. The result can be a displaced spiral fracture of the lower part of the upper arm, near the elbow. The really bad news is this can only be treated by open reduction and

33

internal fixation. In other words, you need an operation involving pins to keep the arm straight and in place while it heals.

I inspected the young man's limb and saw that there was a deformity in the middle of his upper arm. It certainly looked broken. He couldn't move it properly and he yelped when I touched it.

'So, you were arm-wrestling… and then what happened?' I asked.

'Well, it went crack,' he said, 'and he beat me.' He looked at a spiky-haired youth who was standing there nodding and grinning.

I put the lad's arm in a sling and offered him entonox, which he gladly accepted. Then we packed him into the ambulance with one of his mates. No doubt the rest of them carried on with their arm-wrestling competition when we left.

I assumed that was that - the one, freak, pub game injury I'd see in my entire career. Wrong. I attended an almost identical incident the other day - the only real difference was that this time they'd been drinking Magners. We were called to a bar, and the chap in question was already outside, staggering around and moaning in pain, when we arrived. He was being supported by a mate in an Arsenal shirt and I could see the pain on his face as he climbed into the back of the ambulance. His arm was cradled against his chest and he was reluctant to have it inspected.

When I eventually looked at it, I found a number of deformities in the upper arm. He had fractured his humerus in at least two places; the bone was protruding and pushing against his skin - every tiny movement made him scream in agony. Entonox wouldn't touch this level of pain.

'So, what happened?' I asked.

'I was arm-wrestling a mate in the pub when I suddenly felt it go,' he said.

Arsenal boy piped up. 'Yeah,' he said, with a chuckle. 'We heard the crack from the back of the pub. It was really loud.'

The young man whimpered in agreement; I offered him morphine and he gratefully accepted it.

We took him to hospital and he was delivered to the x-ray department within minutes. When I checked back on him a few hours later, he was sitting on a bed awaiting surgery. I didn't think his earlier alcohol-fuelled bravado was worth the pain he now faced.

I decided to look into this and found an article in the *Journal of Bone and Joint Surgery*. (It's not like I keep it lying by my bedside.) There was a piece inside which cited a study carried out in the Department of Orthopaedics at the University Hospital in Hartlepool in which the mechanisms involved in spiral fractures were investigated. They explained how strong internal rotational forces applied to the humerus cause these particular breaks; the resultant fractures are also found in those who use extreme muscular torsion to throw javelins, baseballs and even hand grenades, apparently. Those mechanical arm-wrestling devices you find in cheap amusement arcades have led to a few of these injuries over the years. It sounds funny, but it's actually a really nasty injury. Apart from the pain and the need for surgery, permanent nerve damage can occur.

Apparently, some lunatic has now invented a new game called 'Shocking Arm Wrestling'. It offers the same thrills and spills as conventional arm-wrestling, except that the contenders wear special gloves that deliver electric shocks to the losers. The website boasts that the shock is 'fairly hefty' and warns that it will continue until the pressure is taken off. *"The potential punishment for losing really does inspire you to make sure you're the winner,"* it says. *"After all, it's only the loser that ends up shocked!"*

I guess we were all young once.

MATERNITY

ONE thousand women a day call 999 and say, 'I need an ambulance... I'm about to give birth!'

OK, it's not 1,000, and I don't know how many it is, but it's a lot. It's TOO MANY.

Let's get one thing straight: if you suddenly find yourself in labour, or you have a genuine reason to think things are going wrong, call us, *please*. We're delighted to come out if a mum-to-be is in trouble.

But if you just want a lift to hospital, make your own way there.

Impending childbirth is one of the most common reasons for an ambulance being called when there is no real emergency involved. Some mothers just abuse the system, and we end up being asked to take them in because they haven't got the money for a taxi. Well, I sympathise with anyone who is short of money, but it's not as though motherhood - generally - creeps up on you. Most people have quite a few months' notice. I'll never forget the words of one midwife to the pregnant woman we had wheeled into maternity with plenty of time to spare: 'You've had nine months to save up for a cab!'

As I say, sometimes things do go wrong in pregnancies. According to the baby charity, Tommy's, one in four UK women will suffer a miscarriage; almost everyone in pre-hospital care will have experienced a call to a female of childbearing age who is complaining of abdominal pain and bleeding from the vagina (PV). The diagnosis is often confirmed to both patient and carer alike when there is a discharge containing foetal material.

On one freezing night shift I found myself attending to a woman who had miscarried and was bleeding PV.

PV. 'Per vaginam' is Latin for 'from the vagina' and is often followed by the word bleed to describe bleeding from that particular area. Since the vagina is an orifice leading to a body cavity, any bleeding from it must be taken seriously (unless, of course, it is part of the normal non-conceptual menstrual cycle). A PV bleed during pregnancy may indicate a complication. Similarly, 'PR' is 'per rectum' - 'from or through the rectum'. Again, this is often followed by the word bleed to describe bleeding from that particular area. The rectum is also an orifice leading to a body cavity, so any bleeding from it must be taken seriously (unless it is nothing more than piles or small blood vessel ruptures caused by straining). A PR bleed can indicate disease (such as cancer) or internal haemorrhage.

Her abdominal pain had prompted her to call an ambulance and we took her to hospital. Later on, in the early hours of the morning, my crewmate and I were called back. We found the same woman. She was standing at her door, in tears and fumbling through her handbag. She looked up when we arrived and I got out and asked her what was wrong. She seemed confused and distressed. She was cold, alone and still bleeding, and she was passing little clots of blood onto the doorstep.

She had been sent home by the doctor and told to wait until everything fully discharged from her body. This is standard procedure: sadly, there is little else that can be done.

As we stood there in the chill night, she continued to rummage through her bag in despair, telling me that she could still feel herself bleeding 'down there'. She had lost her door key and couldn't get into the house.

We took her into the warm ambulance and she asked me to collect up the discharged material from her path. 'I just would like to have it,' she said.

I didn't understand why at first, but I went outside again and started picking up what I could. It was dark and I couldn't quite see everything on the ground, so I got my torch and went back to the door and when I shone the light onto the path I found the last few lumps of congealed blood. I turned to go but as I did I caught sight of something else: the light had flashed across a grey-white form on the ground. I knelt down for a closer look and saw that it was the foetus. It was about the size of a fingernail, perfectly formed with tiny bud limbs and two black dots - the eyes. I'd never seen one for real this close up but it was unmistakable. I knew I had to pick it up because it couldn't stay where it was.

I went back for a new clini-waste bag. 'Have you found anything?' said the woman, as I reached into the back of the ambulance.

I couldn't lie - she would have known instinctively - so I told her I'd found her baby.

'Can I see it?' she asked. 'Only, I'd like to have it.'

I nodded and went to see if I could pick the fragile little thing up. I couldn't, it was sticky and difficult to handle without causing damage. Then, almost as if it had been placed there for me, I saw a stick of chewing gum, complete in its wrapper, a foot or so away from the foetus. I used this gently to lift the lifeless little thing up and into my yellow bag. I took it over to the ambulance and asked the woman if she was absolutely sure she wanted it. She said she was.

I unfolded the bag a little and showed her it. There was no new emotion but she stopped crying. I saw resignation on her face; perhaps even the start of closure.

I called my Control to get advice about leaving this woman with no means of getting into her house. I couldn't just abandon her and she had told us she didn't want to go back to hospital because she felt they didn't care. As I waited for a response my colleague told me that the woman had found her

38

keys - they were in her bag all along, she had been too distraught to see them.

We took her back to the house, let her in and sat with her as she gathered herself together again. I placed the foetus in an empty spice jar, at her request. 'I'll bury it,' she said. She was still all alone in the house and this was going to be something she would deal with and live with herself. Her husband hadn't come home and she had no support, only the lost faces of two ambulance paramedics; that was of little comfort to her; I thought.

Before we left, I got her some inco pads so she could put them on her bed sheets. I walked back into the house and found her crying quietly to herself. I held her hand and said, 'I'm so sorry.' I didn't know what else to say or do.

We left her to do what she thought was right and I pondered the emotional horror that miscarriage can be for women. It's hard for a man to imagine the pain they must feel, I think.

* * * * *

My first encounter with a traumatic complication of childbirth came without warning. We received a call by radio for a 25-year-old pregnant female who was giving birth in the back of a car on a residential street. After all the details were taken, the single most important piece of information was added. The baby was a breech; it was being born feet first. Any breech birth is dangerous for the baby, because it's coming out feet first and that means that the shoulders and arms will get stuck in the birth canal. If this happens, the baby will asphyxiate as it lodges in the canal. It's ready to take its first breath, but when it does so it finds its mouth is surrounded by blood, birth fluid and meconium (baby faeces, basically). It ingests that combination and drowns. And this case was the worst kind of breech: this baby was 'front up' and was hanging out of its mother by its neck.

As we approached the street, I saw the car parked with its hazard lights flashing and both rear doors open wide. A man was walking around from one door to the other - there was no real sense of urgency. He didn't look at us. I don't know if he even noticed us there.

I got out of the ambulance as soon as we parked up and went to the rear of the car. I saw a woman crouching on her hands and knees in the back seat. She was completely naked from the waist down and she was crying in pain. There was a small, grey baby literally hanging out of her, suspended by its neck, the body facing forward. It was a little boy. His head was still fully inside his mum's vagina. The scene was bloody and noisy.

I supported the baby's body so that the weight was off its neck and, with the help of the man, who was her husband, tried to get the head released by stretching the vaginal opening. I told the woman to push but she could not understand English and was very frightened. I asked her husband to go to the other side of the car and talk her through what I was doing and what I wanted her to do for me.

My crewmate was gathering the equipment I would need and a second ambulance arrived. The paramedic from this crew assisted me with my efforts to get the baby's head out of the birth canal, but it was proving difficult and the woman was losing the energy to push. Every time she tried the head would begin to appear but then she would give up, exhausted, and it would disappear back inside her. This was very frustrating for all concerned.

At one point, I felt the baby take a breath inside his mother. He moved his limbs and struggled feebly as he tried to escape for air. A flood of mucus and meconium escaped and I knew the baby was in serious danger. I used suction to clear as much of the fluid away from inside the vagina as possible, but it was an uphill battle.

I continued to struggle to release him. The mother was screaming in pain and providing very little effort to the push he needed. I couldn't just rip him from her and I considered what to do. A midwife was needed urgently; the woman would probably need to have incisions made to widen the opening for her baby but there was a delay in getting one to scene, so I had to think about the problem with my colleagues.

As we tried to plan what to do, I felt the baby breathe deeply again, struggle for a few seconds and then go limp in my hands. I didn't feel him move again after that.

The midwife arrived and began to help us with the delivery. It took a further few minutes but she applied as much pulling force as she dared, and with an extra hard push from the mother the baby was free. It had been trapped for over fifteen minutes and he was lifeless in my arms.

We rushed him to the ambulance, continuing our resuscitation attempts. He looked like a tiny rubber doll: every time I pushed down on his chest, his wee arms sprang up. I knew that what I was doing was pointless; I remember thinking, *Why am I doing this? Why don't I leave this poor little thing alone, instead of standing here compressing his ribs and abusing his body even more?*

I kept going all the way to hospital but I was looking down at a lost cause. Newborn babies' eyelids are always closed when they die - this is not always the case with adults, their eyes are usually open or half-open - and they look like they are sad. That's my abiding memory of this little boy: he looked as though he knew he'd nearly made it and was sad that he hadn't.

They lifted him onto a trolley covered in a crisp white sheet and they wheeled him away, a tiny dot of extinguished life that had never seen the outside world.

I felt deeply saddened for his mother. She'd endured a long, agonising experience, and had lost her son at the end of it.

I brought that home with me and I sat and I welled up. I was on my own and I sat there for hours, thinking about that baby. He had been alive when I got there. I'd felt him take his last breath. If we had been able to get him out, he would have lived. He died because we couldn't get him out. He had drowned inside his mother as I held him.

I wrote it all down in my diary, as a way of exorcising it. And for ages afterwards, every call we got for a maternity job, I didn't want to go to it. Sod's law, it just seemed that everyone in north London was having a baby at around that time. No kidding, there was one a day. If I was on the FRU, I'd absolutely dread the message coming up on my screen - especially if it read, *'Complicated birth'*. I would start worrying: *What do I do if this goes wrong, or that happens?* I just didn't want that responsibility, and I found myself driving to the calls dreading knocking on the door, hoping that the ambulance would get there ahead of me, or with me so that I could have back-up.

* * * * *

Eventually, the score was evened out for me.

I was working with a female friend and colleague on a night shift when we received a call to a 23-year-old pregnant female, 'delivery imminent'.

Butterflies. Panicky feeling. At least I wasn't alone.

A first responder was on scene when we arrived. He told us that the woman's waters had broken and she was lying on the floor awaiting the birth. The woman's family were around but they didn't know what to do, so it was going to be up to us to help her. We gave her entonox for the pain and prepared to move her to the ambulance, but she began to push and when I asked if she felt like bearing down she said she did, so I knew we had run out of time. She was wearing shorts so I told her husband to remove them. As soon as they were off we could see the baby's head.

> **PAY.** I love my job, despite the occasional moments of heartbreak. But our rates of pay aren't great. A trained paramedic like me earns around £20,000 a year basic (about £1,000 a year more than an EMT), though there are additional earnings, for London weighting and unsocial hours etc, that mean you can boost this to around £30k (gross).

We positioned ourselves for an imminent delivery. It took no more than three good pushes for the baby to come out. I checked his colour, airway and breathing (although he was crying now, good and strong) and confirmed his sex. I wrote down the time of delivery and then we got with drying him and clamping the cord.

My colleague had never cut a cord before, so she was given the honour. (Umbilical cord is very tough, so it took a few attempts to cut through it properly.) Once that was done, all that remained was the delivery of the placenta, which had yet to materialise after 15 minutes. The placenta is attached to the wall of the womb and it should come out naturally with secondary contractions. If it doesn't, that dead tissue is going to cause problems for the mother. There can also be massive bleeding if it comes away before it's ready, because it will tear away the wall of the womb. That happens a lot, and we can administer drugs to help with it. This was proving less straightforward than the birth itself. The first responder left to attend another call and my colleague and I waited for the midwife to arrive. It actually took two hours for the placenta to show up - two hours of real concern, during which I had a running discussion with the hospital about whether we should bring her straight in and I tried to get the woman to pant and push to discharge it.

After a lot of coaxing and pushing by the woman on the floor, her secondary contractions started and a couple of minutes later the afterbirth was out. The bleeding was controlled and the woman was in good shape, even after the prolonged finale.

She was happy, too; her baby was yowling at the top of his lungs, sounding very healthy indeed.

The midwife arrived ten minutes later. She checked both baby and mother, pronouncing them well. Then I assisted with the last job on scene, stitching up the woman's perineum, which had torn during the birth.

I was happy with this call; it helped give me closure after my horrendous ordeal with the breech a while earlier. I still have a photo, taken by my colleague with the woman's permission, of the little group involved at that birth: me, my colleague, the mum and her baby. It's a happy, smiley memory.

Sometimes even the short distance between a home address and the hospital maternity unit can be too much for an expectant mother. My first Born Before Arrival (BBA) happened so quickly that I barely had a chance to take it all in. I was working with a crew who had just driven a few yards from the patient's home when she suddenly had the urge to bear down. Her waters had broken earlier and we had been called because she felt the birth was imminent. How right she was.

She lay on the trolley bed and my colleague inspected her. The baby was 'crowning', so the top of its head was visible. The woman was moaning in pain and biting hard on the entonox mouthpiece. There was going to be no time for a midwife or another ambulance, so I got the maternity kit and prepared to assist with the delivery.

My colleague coached the woman to breathe and the baby was delivered within two minutes of the appearance of its head. It came out along with a gush of blood and fluid - a lot of fluid. The ambulance floor was awash with it.

The woman screamed in pain as the baby came and then the baby joined in. We were parked up on a residential street close to her home, so the neighbours must have thought we were murdering her. Hopefully the sound of a baby crying helped put their minds at ease.

After the cord was cut and the afterbirth delivered we took them both to the maternity unit. We used our lights and sirens and got to the hospital in a few minutes, much sooner than waiting for additional help.

I ran into the unit with the newborn and the mother followed on the trolley bed. She was weak and exhausted. It took us an hour to clean the ambulance up after that delivery. She wasn't a particularly large woman but she'd held an awful lot of fluid.

A more traumatic BBA was described on my mobile data terminal (MDT) as 'Baby down toilet'. As unambiguous as the call descriptor was, I was still activated on my own for this job with a request to 'report on arrival'. You'd have thought the mother and baby needed more support than just one paramedic, and you'd have been right.

When I got on scene I had to find the address among the myriad identical apartments (not unusual) and then take the lift to the top floor (not unusual either) to the flat in question. I knocked and a man appeared at the door. I was hurried inside and I could smell the location of the problem before I saw it. In a little bathroom a woman was sitting on the toilet, wailing in pain. The man went in, spoke to her (she spoke no English) and then pointed to the floor on the other side of the toilet.

'Is that the baby?' I asked.

'Yes.'

'Is it breathing?'

'I think so.'

God, I hope so, I thought.

45

He moved out of the room and swept his two little sons aside. They had been hanging around the doorway watching this mishap unfold but they seemed completely unfazed. I went in, reassured the lady (with no effect) and then looked down at the floor where the man had pointed. There was a new-born baby lying on its back, umbilical attached, grey as hell - but moving.

It was a girl, and as I watched she seemed to go limp. Quickly, I checked her airway and stimulated her to move and prove that she was breathing. She was: so far, so good. I opened my maternity pack and as I did so a colleague walked through the door. I was very happy to see him.

With his help, I covered the baby and cut the cord - only then could we deal with mum's problem, whatever that was. The FRU desk decided to call me just then (they often seem to do so at the most delicate moments) to ask if I needed any other support. I requested another ambulance in case mum and the baby needed to be taken to hospital separately.

The situation was smelly, messy and noisy but not life-threatening. As far as I could see. The woman had gone to the toilet when she felt the urge to push down. She opened her bowels and, simultaneously, gave birth. The baby fell into the toilet head first. The new-born girl was left in the water of the toilet bowl, covered in faeces until her father had plucked her out and put her on the floor, minutes before I arrived. The woman had made no attempt to do this. The umbilical must have been pulled violently as a result of all of this, and she was now in pain and possibly bleeding behind the placenta, which had yet to appear.

When I wrapped the baby up and handed her to the mother she rejected her immediately. She wouldn't even look at her. She just sat there and wailed. Neither would she let me inspect her, so I asked my female colleague on scene to do it for me. I left the bathroom and went to check on the baby again.

Another ambulance crew arrived and I requested a midwife, too. The woman was going nowhere until the extent of her injuries could be ascertained. My female colleague had confirmed that there was no obvious bleeding, but that didn't rule it out and I had a drug available if needed to stop any serious haemorrhage. But you feel a lot more comfortable with a midwife taking charge, so I left the two crews on scene and drove to the maternity wing of the receiving hospital to pick up the on-call midwife. I rushed her back to the scene and she went to work - job done.

I was able to leave the flat with a sense of having done some good. The woman had been given Entonox for her pain and the baby had begun to colour up nicely. She had ten fingers and ten toes and they all moved, so I was quite happy.

I've delivered or helped to deliver a number of babies in my career, and I'm fine with that. It's the complicated calls I don't like - the responsibility of safely delivering a new life is much more wearing than trying to save an old one.

SUICIDAL TENDENCIES

My colleagues and I get close-up to emotional crises. We all get to see the raw edge of life in this job and suicides, successful or not, are one aspect that none of us relishes dealing with.

My first experience with a suicidal adult came whilst I was still working my way through my degree. I was on the road whenever I had the time to do some paid work with the ambulance service and had started a run of nights when a call for a 'suicidal male' came in.

He was standing on an eighth floor ledge outside the bedroom window of a hotel room, threatening to jump. It was four o'clock in the morning and this was one of London's poshest hotels. If he jumped, the publicity would be extensive and it would not be good.

I stood far below him in the inner quadrant of the building; rooms in this part of the hotel faced each other around a large square and there were plenty of wide-awake guests peering from behind curtains and leaning out for a closer look. At any moment, I expected to hear someone in a room near to the suicidal man open their window and yell, 'For God's sake, jump and let us all get some sleep!'

Until now, the shift had been slow and relatively routine; drunk after drunk until the early hours and then medical emergencies at a steady pace. A call like this could go either way and it was too early in the morning for lucid thought, so I hoped he would see sense and go back into his room.

The London Fire Brigade was already on scene and a couple of police officers were in his room attempting to talk him back to *terra firma*. He wasn't budging, and I noticed that he was standing on a thin ledge which pitched down at something like a 45 degree angle. He was dressed in light clothes, but his feet were bare and probably a little sweaty owing to the grip required for such a precarious position. It wouldn't take much for him to slip and go over accidentally, never mind to leap off.

I looked below him. If he went, he was going to land on the angled glass and metal roof of the restaurant below. Which would be messy. I thought about what I'd do if he fell. There was next to no chance of him surviving - he was 100 feet up. I wasn't worried about having to go down and deal with the aftermath, but I was concerned about having to witness it. That sort of thing makes my skin crawl.

> **MISTAKES. We all make them, and I'm the same as anyone else. I've cocked things up, but - fortunately - it hasn't affected the outcome. Of course, when we get something wrong it can have disastrous consequences. If I put a tube down someone's throat incorrectly, it will kill them, and I will lose my job and professional registration instantly - there is no such thing as an honest mistake if you screw up when intubating a patient.**

My crewmate had wandered off, and now he came back.

'Apparently he's very well-off,' he said, rather stating the obvious. Rooms here were hundreds of pounds a night, even 15 years ago. 'He's fallen in love with a business colleague, but when he told him the colleague rejected his advances.'

The rich man hadn't taken this at all well, and had climbed straight out of the window. The colleague had immediately called 999, and here we were.

I looked up again at the man, far above, teetering on that acutely-angled, narrow ledge, alternately crying and shouting. He was edging away from the window and then back again, almost casually, as though he was on the ground. It seemed to me that his mind wasn't quite made up - I suppose he'd have gone by now if it had been - but it was clear that he was very likely to fall and die accidentally if he kept this up. His screams of despair and anguish grew louder, and soon every guest in the vicinity was awake. More lights shone out of bedroom windows, illuminating the spectacle. The police officers were still trying to coax him back into his room; one of them was leaning out of the window and I could hear the conversation to-ing and fro-ing between him and the potential suicide. It really looked and sounded hopeless and I waited for the inevitable fall that would result in the instant and grisly death of a man right in front of my eyes. Light butterflies of anticipation fluttered in my stomach; I was nervous about what I was possibly about to see.

Almost an hour into the drama, the policeman who was leaning out of the window persuaded the man to come closer; as he slowly sidled towards the window, the copper and his colleague suddenly grabbed him by the legs and waist. He was pulled back inside his room with little fuss. The whole thing was so quick that the suicidal man had no time to react.

He was brought down to us and we took him to hospital. He cried all the way and looked utterly beaten and hopeless. He had, of course, been drinking heavily, but it looked to me as though he was an emotional wreck long before the alcohol convinced him to kill himself. I left him in a cubicle with an unsympathetic police guard and a less than enthusiastic medical team at hand. Attempted self-harm brings few tears to long-suffering NHS staff.

My main feeling was one of relief. Unlike some of my colleagues, I've yet to see someone jump or fall to their deaths. I know it's coming, though, and while I don't mind seeing dead people any more I really don't want to witness the act.

Alongside my relief, there was some anger. People who commit suicide cause a lot of turmoil, to their families and to the people - like me - who come along and clean up after them.

* * * * *

Of the 34 bridges crossing the Thames, the handful in central London are the favoured by the lonely and desperate who want to end it all. Stand on Westminster Bridge, say, with the lights of the Palace of Westminster to your right and the chimes of Big Ben in your ears: launch yourself off there and you'll drop almost a hundred feet before you hit the water, and there's a good chance that will kill you.

Over the years, I've been called to most of these bridges or to the river bank for suspected and confirmed suicide attempts. Once, I got there and the guy was actually sitting on the edge of the concrete, feet dangling, threatening to go over. There were already police on scene watching this young guy looking down at the icy water of the Thames and contemplating his immediate future. He had been caught here before, I was told, and had a long history of psychological problems.

He was eventually 'talked down' and I was asked to take him to hospital. During the journey, I tried to talk to him. 'So why do you want to kill yourself?' I asked.

He looked at me with dead eyes and a face drained of emotion. 'What have I got to live for?' he said. 'Nothing. You're taking me to hospital, that's fine. As soon as I get out I'll try again. Maybe next time...' He left it hanging in the air. I wasn't sure if he was bluffing, but I never saw him again.

A luckier young man was dragged out of the river one night after dropping from London Bridge into the winter water with his rucksack on his back. He'd downed a couple of bottles of champagne and had been seen sitting on the edge of the bridge by a number of witnesses. Then he'd simply slipped off and fallen in. Nobody knew whether he'd meant to fall or not. The police had been called, too, and we'd all raced down there to try and find him. All we knew was he was in the water somewhere downstream of where he had gone in. By now, he'd been in for 20 minutes; it was December, and cold, and that would normally be enough to finish you off, so I wasn't hopeful. Then a police officer called: the guy had been seen floating serenely under Southwark Bridge, on his back, with a peaceful look on his face. He must have been admiring the night sky.

We fished him out a few minutes later. He was alive but very cold and dazed by his experience. Well, either that or he was just too drunk to know what he had done. He'd been saved from drowning by the large amount of air that was in his rucksack. It had kept him above the water long enough for a successful rescue to be carried out. A very lucky young man.

Almost unbelievably, these days we are increasingly called out to suicidal children. I'm not saying it never happened before, but it does seem to be on the rise: Childline says the number of calls it received from kids planning to kill themselves rose by 14% in 2006 and it now takes more than 1,000 such calls annually.

My first experience with this was when I was called to attend a 'child on ledge, threatening to jump'. The child in question was a 12-year-old girl and she was standing on her bedroom window ledge looking down at the police and fire service personnel gathered 20 feet below. If she jumped or fell she would hit concrete, nothing soft in between would break her fall.

She, too, was pulled in by a police officer, a WPC, who talked her out of the mindless thing she was contemplating. Once she was settled down (she was very emotional) it was my crewmate and I who had to continue the necessary care. Her mother and brother had been sitting in the front room as the situation developed outside. They had both been told to stay where they were until the girl had been rescued. I'd anticipated tears of joy and hugs all round after the girl was brought back in, but that didn't happen. Instead, she began accusing her mother of neglecting her and physically abusing her - she stood in the front room shouting in her mum's face about how much she hated her and that she was the reason she wanted to kill herself.

The woman on the sofa sat and cried as her daughter released this tide of venom onto her and I felt very sorry for her, regardless of the accusations made by the young girl. It was clear she didn't want her mother accompanying her to hospital, so the WPC travelled with us. The child was quiet and reluctant to answer any questions during the journey; I thought at first it might be because I was male, but the WPC had no better luck. She wasn't interested in unlocking her emotions and that was a bad start in terms of treatment and future care. I left her feeling pretty down about her chances: I'd have put money on her trying it again, maybe simply in search of some attention from strangers. One day, she might accidentally succeed.

Sometimes, tragically, it isn't a 'cry for help', it isn't an accident and the police aren't on hand to effect a dramatic last-second rescue.

We were called to a 'male, suspended' at a house a few miles off. The journey would take ten minutes on blue lights. When we arrived, the police and a Fast Response Unit paramedic were already on scene. The paramedic shook her head at us as we pulled up. This gesture meant that it was a non-starter of a job, either because it was not as given or because the patient was dead.

'He's inside,' she said. 'A young lad. Dead in his bedroom.'

He had been found by his parents earlier and they had called an ambulance in the mistaken belief that he could be saved, although they had not attempted resuscitation themselves. In fact, when I looked at the call notes later, I saw that they had 'refused to resuscitate'.

We went into the house and found him lying on the floor of his little bedroom. He had been pulled from the bed by his parents when they discovered him and was now on his side, almost in the recovery position, one arm across his chest and one leg raised slightly. Those limbs were still rigid with rigor mortis and that told us a lot about how he had been positioned when he died. His dad looked at me and said, 'Can't you do something for him, then?'

Of course, I couldn't. There's a tremendous feeling of helplessness, but there are limits to our skills.

He was only 19. 'He was right as rain when he got in last night,' said his mother. 'Everything seemed normal. He took himself off to bed without any fuss and that was the last time we saw him alive.'

I looked at the body. At some point, it seemed, he'd placed a plastic bag over his head and suffocated himself. He hadn't struggled much by the looks of things; his body was in a position of sleep, almost as if he had died whilst lying peacefully on his side. I don't know if I could just settle down for a kip with a plastic bag denying me oxygen and life, even if I wanted to kill myself. I'm sure instinct would kick in, and that I'd end up trying to tear the damned thing off my face - but then I've never tried to kill myself, so I may be mistaken. Whatever, in this case there was absolutely no sign of such a struggle taking place. Maybe he had sedated himself with drugs and alcohol prior to placing the bag over his head. Maybe he had resolved not to try and save himself, however powerful the urge. There was no suicide note and he'd arranged things in his bedroom as if he intended to get up the next day as normal. His clothes were laid out ready for the morning and he'd been in the middle of some work on his computer; there was paperwork lying around it. He did have problems with depression, according to his mum. 'I don't know,' she said. 'Maybe he *has* been a bit more unhappy than usual recently.'

I found both parents strangely unemotional under the circumstances. Maybe the shock had numbed them. His father had discovered him first. No attempt had been made to breathe for him or compress his chest. He'd just pulled his son's body to the floor, removed the plastic bag and put it in the rubbish bin. I couldn't understand why he felt he needed to do that. He had to rummage in the rubbish again to bring it out for the police to see. It was a strange call.

> **HAVING A GO. I have taken calculated risks with patients, people who are in very grave danger of dying imminently, where it could have gone the other way, and I've been criticised for that. My attitude is, if the circumstances are right, you *must* have the courage to try anything. If the patient dies that is a tragedy, but if they die and you've tried everything - instead of sitting back and watching - you can look at yourself in the mirror.**

I've had a fair few strange calls, and as I'm curious and investigative by nature that suits me just fine.

I was asked to attend a hanging in one of London's parks. It was cold and foggy and the call came in in the wee small hours. I set out hoping I wouldn't be the first to come across the body. I don't like hangings; it's a creepy way for someone to kill themselves and the face tends to be contorted and grotesque and screaming at you, like you're to blame for its woes. Luckily, I didn't have to get too near this one. When I drove into the park there were a number of other crews already on scene, as well as the police.

I walked toward the area where they were milling about and saw a man dangling like a sick Christmas ornament from the middle branches of a tree. It was quite surreal. He was obviously dead. I've seen a number of hangings. It's comparatively common - Government stats show that it's the most common means of suicide for men (women prefer to poison themselves) - but it was the first I had seen where the act was carried out in public.

He had been found by police because, as they patrolled the deserted service road, they had come across a heavy litter bin which had been lugged into the middle of the asphalt. One of them had got out to move it and had spotted our man dangling lifeless from the tree nearby. They surmised that he might have dragged the bin there as a sort of marker, to attract attention so that he would be found after he'd done the deed. It's even possible that he wanted to be found *trying* to kill himself. If so, unfortunately, fate wasn't on his side.

I stood watching and shivering as he was cut down. He'd chosen the quietest, coldest, foggiest night of the year on which to do away with himself, and it was an eerie and spooky spectacle. Bizarrely, it flitted through my mind that, not too long ago in the past, the sight of a person hanging from a tree in a public place would have been quite normal. Local children would have stood under the corpse and chucked things at it, no doubt.

One bizarre attempted hanging happened on a busy road in north London. I was asked to check on a man who had tried to hang himself from a speed camera and was now fitting. It was a couple of miles away and when I arrived the ambulance crew was on scene and already dealing. The man had bought himself a brand new step ladder, taken it to the camera, pulled a sign over his chest proclaiming how unfair Britain was, gone up the steps, chucked over a ready-noosed rope, covered his head with a brown hood (execution-style) and prepared to step off into oblivion.

Luckily for him, two police officers happened by and casually asked him if he was OK. As he replied he toppled over and began to hang in his (very well-tied) noose. The quick-thinking cops grabbed him and eventually got him down. Now he lay on the pavement, not talking to anyone and being treated for a suspected neck injury. It was a strange call and I have no doubt that he intended to kill himself; everything was too well thought out... except for the possibility that two police officers would stop for a chat mid-suicide; inconvenient, to say the least.

For some reason, there are a lot of suicides in the City. Wealthy people with no apparent problems just throw themselves from buildings, and they rarely leave notes. Not that long ago, a colleague of mine went to one where the guy was in a restaurant, 25 floors up, and he just went to the window and stepped out. The eye witness account was quite horrific. It was daylight, and the guy landed on the roof of a bus. A witness said that, at the moment just before he hit the bus, he let out a little yelp. Normally, people don't make a noise when they jump: I think in this case the guy realised, right at the last second, that death was coming fractionally earlier than he'd thought. They said the usual things about him - he was a happy-go-lucky, well-paid, popular man. No one could understand it.

Of course, the act of suicide may be a dramatically impulsive thing. Many of us will admit to thinking about jumping or falling from a height. When you're on a cliff top, or in some high viewing area, don't you think, for a moment or two, about what it would be like to pitch yourself over and just... fall. Or is that just me?

'One-unders' are good examples of possible 'impulse' suicides. 'One-under' is the term we use for a person who has jumped in front of a train. In London it's a shockingly common way for people to kill themselves, common enough that London Underground has a special 'Therapy Unit' to help drivers with the stress and trauma of seeing it happen. The emotional shock can radiate way beyond the death of the person doing the leaping. London Underground employee Dan

Kuper, writing in *Notes from Underground*, says: *'The drivers take the brunt of the trauma, frequently - ridiculously - blaming themselves for not stopping in time. Each takes it differently, of course, but quite a few never drive a train again, suffering nightmares and flashbacks for months.'*

The thing is, you can pop yourself in front of a speeding tube in almost any station in the capital; only a few, between Westminster and Stratford on the Jubilee Line, have safety doors to keep people away from the tracks. (Equally, you can be pushed or knocked accidentally - personally, I *never* stand anywhere near the edge of the platform because you can be on the tracks in a millisecond.) Strangely, the majority of such incidents happen underground, despite the fact that only around 45% of the London Underground is actually subterranean. Maybe there are more depressed people inside than outside the City, or maybe it's something about the dark claustrophobia of the Tube.

Many jumpers do not die instantly. The deep underground stations have pits under the tracks. These were designed as drainage gutters, but are now known as 'anti-suicide pits', 'suicide pits' or 'dead man's trenches', depending on how colloquial you want to be. Rather than falling onto the tracks, the person often ends up in the trench, and while very few survive - there is tremendous force involved when something so big hits you at speed - this sometimes prevents them from dying instantly.

As Dan Kuper says, 'How the Tube got its reputation as a good spot for suicides is a mystery. It is a completely stupid choice. A large number of jumpers don't die immediately. Those that are successful often manage because they get themselves crushed between the far wall and the train, instead of on the rails. It is very far from clinical. At the first one-under I attended, the woman was still alive underneath the train, screaming and trying to get up. The image stayed with me for years.'

Picking up the pieces after a 'one under' is never pleasant, and for the individuals who choose to end their lives this way it will be no 'cry for help'. These usually involve a long, drawn-out process like overdose, poisoning, wrist-cutting, that sort of thing. You can't call a leap in front of a fast train a cry for help.

Someone posted a photo on www.Londonlogue.com entitled 'Looking for attention on the Tube'. It shows a young woman, dressed in a jacket and tracksuit, lying inside the suicide pit at the edge of the platform. She has her hood pulled over her head and appears to be in an almost foetal position. She looks determined to stay there. Ironically, if a train had gone over her she would have been unhurt because it would have been too high up to make contact with her, unless she planned to stand up and face it at the last moment. The commenter makes this statement about her:

> She was saved after fellow passengers managed to get staff to stop the oncoming train and switch off the power, after she'd refused their help to get back on the platform.
>
> There are a number of people who get killed by falling or jumping onto the Tube lines every year and the knock on effect for travellers can be a nightmare with lines closed down for long periods. Why turn commuting into a more miserable experience for thousands of people just by showing off and jumping in front of a train?
>
> This woman told police who arrested her 'If not today, I am going to do it tomorrow'. They should say fine, kill yourself if you want, but here's a length of rope and a jar of sleeping pills. Do everyone else a favour and either overdose or hang yourself but don't screw up people's journey home.

A commuter's point of view that may be, but selfish acts on the Underground do, indeed, have a knock-on effect.

I was called to a young drunken man who was pulled out of the pit during a shift near Christmas. He had stepped over the edge accidentally and then laid down for a sleep. He had a head injury and was completely oblivious to the danger he had put himself in. Luckily for him the train was still a few minutes away and Underground staff had been alerted by passengers who witnessed his stumbling stupidity. Railway platforms are no place to be drunk; they should consider banning people from travelling if they are legless.

* * * * *

The one I remember most vividly was my first. It happened at London Bridge station a while back and it ended up being shown in an episode on BBC's *Trauma* programme, a fly-on-the-wall documentary series following emergency crews as they went about their business.

I was working with a colleague on a routine transfer call and had just arrived at the address when this higher priority call came through as a GB.

'One-under at London Bridge, any mobile able to respond please press Priority.'

We pressed the button and got the call. I wasn't at all sure if I wanted it, but then what normal human being looks forward to seeing what a man looks like after a tube train has run over the top of him?

> **GB. General Broadcast. A radio alert which goes out to ALL frontline vehicles (known as mobiles) on a specific channel. The broadcast contains information or requests crews to 'green up' and make themselves available for a call that is queuing. At busy times, GBs are common.**

We got the blue lights on, dodged through the afternoon traffic and were on-scene within a few minutes. A couple of solo paramedics had already arrived and we made our way down the escalators to see what we could do to help. It was hot and noisy and sweaty, but all thought of personal comfort evaporated when we got to the platform. The train had stopped and most of it was inside the tunnel; the last carriage or two was still on at the platform and we could see the activity underneath.

A paramedic was already there, tending to the patient who, incredibly, was still alive. According to witnesses, he had jumped in front of the train (one-unders are usually witnessed, by the poor driver if nobody else) and had been dragged underneath.

His torso had hit the train but his head had failed to make contact. Now he was trapped underneath, with massive internal injuries, affecting his chest and abdomen. Amazingly, he hadn't lost any limbs and he didn't have a mark on his head. He was still breathing and just about conscious. He wasn't talking to anyone, just moaning and groaning softly. My crewmate and I got down and crawled under as far as we could to offer our assistance. The LFB had arrived and they were going to lift the train off the track so that we could slide the man and ourselves out from underneath. Unfortunately, they can only lift the train a few inches off the rails, so it's still a tight and dangerous squeeze on exit.

Another crew had arrived now and a trolley bed and further equipment was being brought down. HEMS arrived; the first thing I knew about it was when I turned around to speak to someone and found myself looking at an orange-suited doctor and a BBC camera. (My butt was the first thing you saw of me on the programme when it aired.)

> **HEMS.** The Helicopter Emergency Medical Service, based at the Royal London Hospital in Whitechapel. They are an elite team of doctors and paramedics who are called to the most serious patients, where difficult entrapment or major trauma is involved. Sometimes they travel by helicopter (during daylight hours) and sometimes in a specially-liveried fast response car. They are activated either directly by Control or by crew request.

We continued to try and untangle the man's body; he was twisted under the train's metal structures and was effectively caught on the bottom with his legs wrapped around a cross bar. As soon as the train was moved and he was freed, I heard yelling and banging around and someone calling for suction. Something had gone wrong. I passed the suction equipment through and the horribly-injured guy was dragged out after a few seconds. He had gone into cardiac arrest.

He was resuscitated on the platform, and a thoracotomy was prepared. This is something HEMS can do but we cannot; it's a hugely invasive procedure that involves cutting holes in the chest at each side and then cutting right across and opening the chest cavity in order to get at the internal organs, particularly the heart, directly. I have never seen anyone survive a thoracotomy, it is just about the most desperate thing you can do, a last-gasp, last hope affair - the sort of risk-taking I talked about earlier. On this occasion, once the holes were put in, resus had become so desperate that the decision was made not to open him up completely. I was bagging the man, and every time I pushed air into his lungs blood would spurt out of the two holes in his side. It wasn't pretty.

As I ventilated him, I looked down at his face. He was well-fed and his clothes weren't begging gear. He didn't look like he had come off the street, he looked as though he had a life somewhere. He had a number of tattoos on his body, including one of the Scottish flag. A fellow countryman.

The resus effort was called off after almost an hour of hard work. There was no way he could be brought back. His internal injuries were significant enough to have caused him to lose almost all of his blood: there was certainly enough of it around that platform. As he was bagged up, I wondered what had driven him to this. I wondered, too, what it had been like. How would it feel to stand on a platform, waiting for the distant rattle and echo of an approaching train, with commuters and tourists chatting away nearby, counting down the final seconds of your life? And what would it be like as you threw yourself onto the track? He'd have been hoping for a sudden despatch, but that's not what he got. He had suffered for some time after being hit by the train, though his plans had eventually come to their terminal fruition. He had achieved what he had set out to do. But why had he done it?

A few weeks after this job, my second call of the night - after a successful resuscitation - was to attend a 'one under' at a central London tube station.

The LFB, police and an ambulance were on scene and a motorcycle solo had travelled with me. A large crowd had gathered outside the station because the evacuation alarm had been activated and the station had been cleared. The crowd made it difficult to get access to the entrance and I had to struggle through the mass of people to get to the gates, which were being guarded by the police and underground staff.

On the platform, a group of medics, police officers, fire personnel and tube staff had gathered. One of my colleagues had volunteered to get under the train with a fireman and they had both climbed down, only to be told to keep still because nobody was sure if the power was off. They both froze where they were, but not before my colleague had checked the man's vital signs and found them to be absent - he wasn't breathing and he didn't have a pulse. He was still lying where he'd been hit, everyone waiting for the Tube staff to verify that the power was off. It's hot and dirty down there and the last thing you need is the additional worry of possible electrocution: two colleagues from my station had previously suffered severe electric shocks under a train after being given assurances that it was safe. They could easily have been killed and this risk is simply not acceptable, especially when the person who jumped may well be dead anyway.

I looked underneath the train and saw a man lying on his side with a large pool of blood around his head. He wasn't breathing at all. He had obviously died of his injuries, but we still had to get under the train to confirm that. We stood on the platform with all the other services, waiting for the word.

Once the all-clear was given, further checks were made but it was obvious the man hadn't survived. The HEMS team arrived just as the two volunteers were climbing out of the pit. I described what we had and the doctor got down to confirm that the man was beyond help. I went in with him and waited until he had done what was necessary.

The body was left where it lay and the train was moved away to reveal it for the police and Coroner to examine. It wouldn't be moved until that had been done, so the platform would remain closed.

Outside, the traffic was building up. Long queues were developing all over the West End, partly due to the sudden increase in taxis flooding the area to carry commuters home, and partly because of some existing road works. The main cause of the chaos, however, was the virtual car-park of emergency vehicles in the area and the forced closure of the roads around the station.

I left the station platform and headed for fresh air. While I was doing the paperwork, a member of London Underground staff approached me and asked if I could take care of a young woman who had been sitting outside the station entrance, crying. I took her to the car and she was soon joined by a friend who had been called to take her home. I decided to take her to hospital, with her agreement, because she was in a very bad emotional state.

During the journey, which was painfully slow due to the heavy traffic, I looked at her in my rear-view mirror. Her face was a mask of deep and painful emotion; she looked haunted, her eyes almost terrified, and she said nothing throughout the journey.

Who was this frightened, scarred young woman? She was the commuter who had been standing next to the man when he had jumped in front of the train.

HEAVY PEOPLE

Heavy people are a pain in the back.

Unfortunately, some of the heaviest people are also our most regular customers. Their weight causes them health problems (which will almost certainly result in an early death), and they often need hospital treatment. So their large frames have to be removed from their tiny flats (on the hundredth floor). By us.

Lifting overweight patients is one of the most common causes of injury in the NHS. Every year, 4,000 nurses are forced into retirement because of back problems, and 5,000 other NHS workers need time off. The majority of such injuries occur when staff in the caring services lift, carry and move patients.

Ambulance service personnel are particularly vulnerable. Many care homes now do not allow their staff to do any lifting or moving of patients; instead they call an ambulance and we come and do it for them. The same applies to domestic carers; we will often be called to a person's home to carry out an 'assist-only'.

When I'm working on the FRU, I don't have to do a lot of lifting. Ambulance crews do that, and some of the weights they need to shift don't bear thinking about. Of course, I offer my help wherever I can; it's important to keep in practice because your back can weaken over time and you'll be caught out one day when it's unavoidable.

I was in an ambulance when a frequent flyer called us out. She had fallen on the floor and couldn't get up. Her front door was open, thanks to a friendly neighbour, and she was hollering from her bedsit for us to 'get a move on'. We walked in and - to our surprise - found her sitting in a chair.

'Did you get yourself up off the floor then?' I asked, more than a little irritated that we had wasted our time.

'I was never on the floor,' she barked back.

'We were called to help you get off the floor.'

'Well, I just want you to move me to my bed.'

This very large woman had called us so that she could be transferred from her chair to her bed. That was it.

I wasn't happy, but I kept a smile on my face, as did my colleague.

During the laborious process of moving her, she shouted orders at us, telling me to do specific things, like move an ornament or bring her a certain item to help her move in a certain way. She had a routine and she was forcing us into it by ordering us about. While it is always necessary to maintain a professional front, inside I really felt like telling her to get on with this herself and pointing out that we had much more important things to do. We spent more than an hour with her as we jostled and shoved her into a position that was 'just right' for her comfort in bed.

I knew this woman would be calling another crew soon after we left. She would need to go to the toilet after all that excitement.

In the end, we do our jobs and we call in support when we feel it's necessary. We use special tools and aids if we can get hold of them, and we have occupational health to hobble to when we get it wrong. But none of that will prevent the problem from getting worse in the near future. Our fat kids are becoming fat adults with fat habits that will not be assuaged by lean advertising and the aspirations of the vegetarian minority.

Being obese, apart from the few with real problems, is often about culture, poverty and ignorance. Alcoholism and fast-food consumption contribute largely to the swelling population of fat folk and the kids who grew up overweight are now indulging in those social evils as part and parcel of their calorie runaway diets. It's probably safer to smoke.

My crewmate and I were sent to another large lady who had fallen out of bed and could not get up again. She was so obese that she couldn't find her own centre of gravity and simply rolled around on the floor gasping and moaning as she attempted to right herself. Her family stood by, unable to help. She was just too heavy: probably somewhere over 25 stones (or 158 kilos, if you prefer).

Usually, on a particularly heavy or awkward lift, another crew can be requested and on more than one occasion I have done this, simply because I knew I'd do my back in if I attempted to do it alone or with just one other person. On this occasion, there were no crews available. My colleague and I had a long look and eventually figured we could get the job done with the right planning.

We lifted her, under a lot of strain, to the edge of the bed and asked her to 'wriggle' her way backwards until she was balanced. Then we swivelled her legs around so that she just fell back onto the bed. Mission accomplished, with a lot of sweating and grunting from us.

A particularly awkward lift requiring two crews involved carrying another lady (who wasn't all that heavy but was unable to move) in a chair over the balcony of her extremely narrow staircase. She had to be lifted above our heads. There were four of us, one at each corner of the chair and she had three floors to go before we could rest. It was a precarious and nerve-wracking transfer, but at no point was she in any danger, we all knew what we were doing and had done it many times before. The patient, however, may not feel as confident.

Older estates have tall buildings with concrete stairwells and no lifts. The worst carrying jobs are the ones involving people with chest pains who live in such buildings. Your back screams in protest as soon as the call comes in, because you know that you're going to have to walk all the way back down those stairs with a patient on a chair. It screams even louder when you see that the patient lives on the tenth floor, weighs 23 stones and has thighs that will overflow and obstruct the smooth movement of the skinny ambulance chair he has to sit in.

I helped a crew on a call when they had a very obese woman to move. She was on the floor of her tiny little front room and she literally filled the area with her sheer mass. Around her were fag ends and junk food packets, crisps and sweets and more than enough chocolate for the whole service to share. She obviously hadn't been paying attention to the Government's healthy-eating lectures.

Her corridor was narrow and she hadn't left the house in years, so this was going to be fun.

Not.

My crewmate and I had to go and get a special vehicle just to take her bulk. It's called the Special Care Baby Unit, or 'SCaBU', and it's wide and uncluttered so was the perfect vehicle to roll her into. We still had to get her off the floor though and for that we used an inflatable device called an ELK. This lifted her slowly up to a level where she could be managed easier. It still took six of us to prise her out of that house and into the ambulance.

Obesity is a real problem in this country. My university dissertation was all about childhood obesity and its potential effects on the NHS, particularly the ambulance service. I could see more young heart attacks, more fat people in high rise buildings (with no lift) and many more job-related injuries, especially back injuries, as a direct result of lifting and moving said fat people. All the ergonomic training in the world won't make any difference to the outcome if the trend in obesity continues, because we're heading for a 50% fat-folk nation.

Almost two thirds of the population of England were overweight in 2004, representing a 400% increase on the past 25 years. Predictions suggest obesity will overtake smoking as the number one cause of premature death. In fact, this could be the first generation of modern times where life expectancy will actually start to fall.

Meanwhile, some of my colleagues will be forced out of the job because of back trouble, some will endure until it becomes impossible to work and some will be smart enough to stay away from dangerous or heavy lifts until they have planned it properly or roped-in more volunteers. I've never heard a crew moan once about helping their pals out in these situations.

Me, I can't stand for long periods without developing a deep lumbar pain which is only relieved when I sit down. I have suffered like this for over ten years now - that's the price you pay for lifting heavy people.

CYCLISTS

London's cyclists can be dangerous, and a lot of them - certainly in the centre of town - flout the law at every opportunity. They zip across pavements, weave in and out of traffic and - worst of all - they think red lights don't apply to them. Why won't they stop like everyone else? Is it too inconvenient? Are they busier or more important than the rest of the population? Do they honestly think they aren't committing or causing any offence? The thing is, they get away with it - while dangerous drivers and speeding motorcyclists can be photographed and tracked down, cyclists can break the law with impunity. There's no way of catching them unless a copper actually sees them at it.

I started spouting off about how dangerous most cyclists can be on my blog in 2006; that year, *The Guardian*'s Matt Seaton reported that only four had been prosecuted in the last 12 months. Four! Anyone who has driven in London will know that's a tiny proportion of the actual offences they commit, which must run into the thousands. In the same piece, Seaton highlighted a school in the city where teachers and parents were up in arms because cyclists kept running a nearby red light and had hit and injured a number of kids.

I've attended the victims of mad cyclists, and I've also had to treat one or two of the perpetrators of this idiocy after they came off worst.

I was called to a 20-year-old who had slammed into a lamp post at full speed in an attempt to navigate his way around traffic. The traffic was moving and he was cutting in and out between cars, which isn't clever. He fell foul of one when it almost clipped him; he lost control and hit the post without braking. He wasn't wearing a helmet and he was lucky not to be killed. As it was, he sustained a nasty head injury and a badly broken collar bone. Obviously, he was in some discomfort but he was stable with no neck pain or other significant injury. There was plenty of blood around from his head wound, but a first aider had rushed out from a nearby office and put a large dressing on it. This Good Samaritan had also offered to secure the man's bike for him while he was taken to hospital. His acrobatic cycling had almost cost him more than a lost Raleigh and he made one sensible comment as I treated him: 'I think I'll take the bus next time.'

As it happened, I had a second cyclist the same day. She, too, got off scot-free, but it could have been horrendous. She'd been behind a large lorry and had tried to nip in between it and the pavement, just to save a few seconds of time. The driver of the truck hadn't seen her, and had effectively driven over her. He'd managed to crush the bike underneath a wheel and caught her under his trailer. Luckily - does 'lucky' describe this? - an alert passer-by had seen it happen and had screamed and waved to the driver. He'd slammed on the anchors and then, under the guidance of the witness, had gingerly reversed a few inches, allowing the trapped woman to free herself without injury. Another second, maybe a second and a half, and she'd have had a 20 tonne truck roll straight over her.

A two car RTC that was caused by the erratic cycling of a man who had tried to dodge in between them as they moved across a junction had me trying to keep the drivers and the cyclist involved apart. They wanted to beat him up and it eventually took the arrival of the police to calm things down. Luckily nobody was seriously hurt, but both vehicles were damaged.

Car drivers aren't innocent, either; I've never had a cyclist die on me but I've been to a few who have gone over the bonnet or bullseyed a windscreen because the driver has cut them up.

Cyclists

During the summer, the traffic police held a free demonstration on safe cycling in which cyclists were invited to come onto Trafalgar Square and park next to a lorry. Then they could climb into the cab of the lorry and see just how invisible they were to the driver if they parked too near his vehicle. The idea was to simulate the stopping behaviour of cyclists when they are at traffic lights (when they aren't running them) and to encourage discussion about the danger they put themselves in.

I spoke to the officers running this demo and they told me that of the very few cyclists who bothered to show an interest, some of them had argued their rights instead of taking in the lesson.

Of course, not all cyclists are mad and more than a few of them do behave properly on the road. But I spent an hour or so one shift counting the number who ran red lights and zipped through active pedestrian crossings - 30 out of 33 I saw broke the law.

DRUGS

The increase in drug abuse in the UK has had a direct and serious impact on the NHS in recent years.

From a purely personal perspective, I find I am dealing with more and more drug-related incidents as time goes on. Many of these calls are to unintentional overdoses; others are the victims of drug crime... the shootings, stabbings and robbery-assaults.

If an overdose has been caused by an opiate, like heroin, I can effectively reverse it and save the patient's life with a drug we carry. I've had to do this many times - I couldn't count how many - and, in the early days, I got the sense of satisfaction that you should get with the recovery of any dying patient. Unfortunately, as the jobs and years passed, that feeling depleted. Nowadays, I tend to feel as if I have been used.

Why? Well, for one thing, no drug user - not a single one - has ever thanked me or my colleagues (as far as I know) for saving their lives like this.

In fact, you usually get the opposite.

This may surprise you, but I've treated heroin overdoses - I'm talking semi-conscious people who are very close to death - and brought them back from the brink... only to have them recover and launch a verbal, even physical, attack on me for ruining their 'fix'. They don't like it when their money has been poured out of their veins.

The drug we use, Naloxone, is usually harmless, though some people can have serious withdrawal symptoms if it is given too quickly. It has only one purpose - to reverse the physical effects of a narcotic - so it's also known as 'Narcan' (Narcotic antagonist). We'll give the drug where we find anyone unconscious with depressed breathing and pinpoint pupils, unless there is another explanation.

As you get more adept at giving this drug, you start to reduce the dose or dilute it, so that you can reverse the life-threatening effects of the heroin without fully awakening the patient. That way, you can keep them 'groggy' enough to handle until you leave them at hospital. This means you keep yourself and your colleague safe and the hospital security staff can deal with any uprising afterwards. They're more equipped for that than we are. Patients who were at death's door an hour or two ago frequently storm out of the Accident & Emergency department in a rage when they realise where they are and what has been done. Again, never a word of thanks.

Sometimes we don't get there in time. Sometimes, no-one could have. I've attended fatalities where people have been found dead with the needle still sticking out of their arm or groin, such was the speed of their demise. They rarely have anyone in the immediate vicinity to mourn for them, except for their addict friends.

I went to a murder scene a few years ago in which the victim had allegedly been killed over a drugs dispute. At first, the call seemed innocuous: 'Strange smell coming from flat, please investigate.' In itself, not that concerning: the last time I went to one of those calls, the householder had simply left their rubbish sacks in the hallway and gone on holiday. Over the weeks, the heat had made everything organic stink and that was what was upsetting the neighbours.

So we made our way to the estate and climbed the stairs to the correct floor. The door to the flat had been forced and was slightly ajar - not much, but enough for us to know that someone had either entered recently, or had left and forgotten to close the door properly. Needless to say, we were very cautious.

I peered into the hallway after knocking several times and getting no reply. 'Hello,' I said. 'Anyone in?'

Still nothing. I leaned further in.

At first I didn't see anything, but then, through a doorway, I saw an arm sticking out. I moved position, squinted, and realised there was a man's body lying on a narrow bed just ahead in the front room, which was also the bedroom. As my eyes adjusted to the different light, I saw his face. He wasn't moving. I was about to go in, but my colleague pulled me back.

'Crime scene,' she said.

Good point; if the guy inside had died suspiciously, the police would confiscate my boots and probably my uniform for their forensics people to pull apart. I didn't fancy having to wait on scene in a white coverall until my DSO showed up to supply me with another uniform, so I stood my ground. That left us with a problem. Somehow, we had to confirm that he was dead and didn't need immediate help. From the doorway, it looked quite obvious; his arm was stiff and very discoloured and I could see that his chest wasn't moving and his face was still. We needed to make sure, though.

We deliberated for a few minutes before we hatched a plan. I put a blanket on the floor of the flat and used it to shuffle into the room while my colleague stayed behind to bring in the police, who had now been called. I approached the man, keeping a very wary eye on the kitchen door, which stood ajar to my left. I didn't know if there was anyone still in here, and we've all seen those horror movies where the unsuspecting minor character gets butchered when he least expects it. I convinced myself that it was safe and looked closely at the man on the bed. He was dead for sure, a definite purple plus. Rigor mortis had set in and he was mottled in blues and greys throughout his body.

He looked strangely at peace, except for the fact that his mouth was open, as if in a final gasp or at some sudden shock. He had a head injury on his right side; his face was badly swollen there and his skull looked deformed. It looked to me as though he had been hit unexpectedly and very hard, and had died instantly as a result. His body hadn't moved from a lying position - you can tell by the staining and pooling of blood, drained by gravity into the lower extremities of the corpse - and he hadn't made any obvious effort to struggle. He couldn't have screamed, either, because none of the neighbours had reported anything unusual.

An ashtray, overspilled with burned out spliffs and cigarettes, was on the floor next to him.

And he had lain here, from the moment the hammer or bat or bar had connected with his skull, for several days. With the door slightly ajar. None of the neighbours even knew what was inside the flat. Nobody - not even the kids living on his floor - had bothered to push open the door to find out what lay inside.

When the police arrived, they interviewed the immediate neighbours but nothing had been seen or heard. The man had a 'friend' who visited regularly but nobody knew who he was or when he was last on the premises.

We lost our blanket of course - it was evidence. But better that than my boots.

Other drug addicts just want to rid themselves of their lives. It's often easier for them than trying to kick the habit. I took a Red Cat A call for an 'overdose, needle in arm, not moving'. It sounded like a classic heroin OD and I was sure this was going to be a messy resus.

I knew the location. It's a hostel for the lost and unlikely-to-recover individuals of society, the drug addicts, alcoholics and ex-cons who inhabit its squalid rooms. They either live alone or, occasionally, with a dog for company.

I arrived to find the people in charge of the place milling around outside, banging on the front door and screaming for someone to let them in. They had locked themselves out. At this point, I thought the call was going to descend into farce.

We got in and I found the man. He was sitting outside his room, and he wasn't dead. He told me that he had injected himself with heroin (at least, he thought it was heroin - it doesn't come with a money-back guarantee) and that he had also taken a load of prescription pills of various colours and types. I checked him over thoroughly and decided that it was actually unlikely he had taken anything at all. I looked up at the battered door to his room: he had taped a note to it reading, 'By the time you read this I will be dead - take care of my dog for me.'

Poignant but pointless, I thought.

The man was generally unpleasant and this 'cry for help' was just the latest of many. There is counselling, advice and structured support out there for guys like him, but some of them just don't care. Drugs do that to people. It's a vicious circle: they take drugs, so they lose the self-interest and self-respect which are vital if they are to improve their lot, so they take more drugs.

I popped my head around his door to say hello to his dog. On the floor, wrapped in a blanket, was a well-mannered and frightened mongrel. I offered him my apologies before I left the scene. I think he understood, although I could still see deep misery in his big brown eyes.

Another overdose took me and my colleague on a journey into a dark and dangerous part of town. There was somebody peering out of a window of the premises we had to enter and none of the lights were on. I decided it might not be a good idea to venture on until we had some reassurance that this wasn't a trap. I get a bit paranoid when things don't feel right. A neighbour came out and assured us that he knew the people inside and that we would come to no harm. And since the police had been called and were on their way, we took the man's word and entered the building.

TRAPS. I've mentioned that we regularly get assaulted and, even more regularly, abused. Less commonly, some people also lie in wait to rob us. They may be after our drugs, our stab vests or the Mobile Data Terminals (MDT) from our vehicles. They make a 999 call and find a good place to hide before either confronting us or getting to our vehicles while we investigate the call. They're wasting their time, however; we don't carry enough drugs to make a robbery worthwhile, our vests are tailor-made, so won't necessarily fit them, and our MDTs are useless without the service software that runs them.

Inside, lying on the grotty floor of an even grottier kitchen, was a teenager. He was unconscious and barely breathing, a large and strong-looking guy who didn't fit the profile of a regular user. *He will soon enough*, I thought. *If he survives*.

The paraphernalia around the room, which included loaded and ready-to-use syringes, told us all we needed to know about his current condition. His skinny, greasy-haired girlfriend cried and shouted uselessly beside him, demanding that he 'get up and behave'. It looked like it was her first time with a heroin overdose; he wasn't getting up any time soon, or ever again if we didn't get a move on.

She turned to us. 'Help him,' she yelled, tears streaking her wild-eyed face. 'Don't let him die!'

'We'll do all we can,' said my colleague as I prepared the IV equipment and got the Narcan out.

It didn't take long to get some of the stuff he needed into his veins, but he didn't respond. There were three of us on scene now; the FRU had just arrived, and the patient was being 'bagged' to keep his breathing rate up while my crewmate and I got ready to move him to the ambulance.

The police turned up. They took one look at the scene and let us get on with our job, temporarily ignoring the incriminating evidence that littered the room. I think they knew better than to upset this apple cart just at that moment. A few minutes later, we'd done all we could for him at the scene.

'You guys ready to go?' one of the officers said.

'Yep,' I said. 'Just give us a minute to get the trolley bed in.'

Once he was on the bed and in the ambulance, I gave him another bolus of the good stuff and watched. He started to come round; he was groggy but becoming more stable. His breathing rate was increasing and his blood pressure was normal.

'Is he alright?' asked the skinny girl.

'He should be now.'

'But he's not awake properly. What's wrong with him?'

'He's a drugged-up idiot,' I almost said. But the words slipped by when I realised he could probably hear me. 'I've kept him a bit sleepy so that he doesn't cause any problems for us,' I said instead.

'He's as gentle as a lamb,' she sobbed. 'He wouldn't hurt a fly.'

I wondered if she knew how many times I had heard that line, especially from the mean owners of meaner dogs.

We took him to hospital and left him in the care of the staff on duty. We were back not long after with another patient, and I wasn't flavour of the month. Our overdosing teenager had woken up after another Narcan injection and had gone crazy in the Resus room. Apparently, he'd abused the nurses, thrown some stuff about and then stormed out, threatening to sue the hospital and the ambulance service for the money he had lost. Gentle as a lamb, eh?

* * * * *

As with our friend above, not all druggies look like hell (though most do). A few weeks back, I was on earlies on the FRU and I was called to an overdosed drug addict who wasn't breathing very well. I went up to the sixth floor of this shabby block of flats in Camden, expecting to find a horrible, disgusting, skinny, spotty drug addict. Instead, lying in the corner of a junkie flat, was a vision of beauty. She was stunning, a slender young woman with long dark hair and big Spanish eyes. But for the needle hanging out of her arm, she might have been asleep.

We brought her round, and I spoke to her.

'How long have you been doing this?' I said.

'About two years,' she said.

I looked around the flat, which was obviously a regular haunt for crackheads and heroin addicts. I strongly suspect she was selling her body for gear. *What the hell are you doing here?* I thought. *There's a life out there, just waiting for you.*

'You've got to stop this, or else one day you will go under and you won't come back,' I said.

She nodded, but she was elsewhere.

This was one of the saddest jobs I've been too. It really depressed me: she was the same age as my son. And it was so bloody *pointless*.

EARLIES. Shifts which start at 6.30am or 7am. They usually present a slower start because people are not yet up and around so they aren't trying to kill themselves by falling, crashing, running into brick walls, arguing with their drunk neighbours or mainlining speed. You get to see daylight and it's safer than working late at night. You might even get breakfast.

One of the strangest drugs calls I attended didn't look like an OD at first; I only found out how the guy had died much later on, when I treated another addict weeks later who just happened to know him. I called this one 'The Mystery of the Dead Man with the Shiny Shoes'.

Life And Death On The Street

I was called to a 'possible lifeless person'. It came from the police and it was the second time they'd asked for one of us to investigate. I was a bit confused: tends to be you're either lifeless or you're not, and the police are pretty good at spotting the difference. I went to the address given but nobody in the street knew what was going on. There were no cops there and nobody had called the Service. An ambulance arrived soon after I did and we hung around while I called it in. Control gave me another, more accurate, address and off we all went.

We drove around the corner and we *still* couldn't find the police or the supposedly lifeless body. I called Control again. As I did so, a motorbike solo paramedic arrived with us; now it was beginning to look like the Service staff meeting. Just as we were all about to quit, a police van came round the corner and stopped, quite casually, in front of my car. The officer got out - no hurry - and said to me and the motorbike solo, 'You want to see it then?'

He took us to a locked gate which we all had to clamber over (it was spiked at the top, so it was a delicate operation) and into an old and derelict factory. This really surprised me: prime real estate, smack in the middle of Central London; the space was worth a fortune.

We went up two flights of stairs, across an open floor maybe 2,000 feet square, and then up another flight of stairs which was barred off by dangling wires and cables (it looked like someone had done this to restrict entry). We then walked across another open area, at the far end of which another PC stood.

He pointed into a small room behind him. I couldn't quite see what was in there but I noticed some personal effects lying around and so I picked up a driving licence. It bore the photo of a young man in his late 20s.

'Is this him?' I asked.

'Yep,' said the standing officer.

Drugs

I went forward and had a look in the room. There was a body on a filthy mattress. He looked like he was asleep, lying on his left side with his legs drawn up slightly. All around us was evidence of rough sleeping and drug use. There was filth and rubbish everywhere - old needles, stained, doss-down mattresses, the discarded detritus of an informal drugs den. But the dead man was wearing a suit, and his black shoes were buffed to almost military standards. He looked healthy and well-fed. There was no needle in his arm.

I clambered over the mattress and stood astride him to carry out the usual examination. I checked his carotid pulse; none. His skin was cold, and as soon as I touched him a fly came out of his mouth. It was probably laying eggs in there. That was enough, really, but I checked for rigor mortis, too, and his limbs were indeed stiff and set in their terminal positions.

There was no sign of any violence. The police had checked, and I double-checked: no, he really did look as though he'd somehow found his way in here, lain down on the mattress and just died in his sleep. A proper autopsy would reveal all, but that would come later, and elsewhere.

It was a mystery: this was no street person, or obvious junkie, so why was he here? It obviously crossed my mind that he'd come here to use drugs, but he looked like a City boy - not a Porsche-driving broker, but certainly someone well-paid and pretty successful, hardly the type to use his gear in a squalid dump like this. Lines of coke in nightclub toilets, yes, but syringes full of H in deserted factories? Maybe I was being naïve, but I didn't think so.

I left the man with the shiny shoes and the watchful police and made my way back outside. I wondered how he'd met his end here. And then I got in the car and got on with my day.

A few weeks later, I was treating another drug addict. We talked about the chances of him dying through drugs, and he said he knew this was a possibility because it had happened

83

recently to a friend of his. In an abandoned factory. His friend turned out to be the shiny-shoed dead man. It's a small world, the drugs world, and - as the big-eyed brunette had shown me earlier - not everyone in it is as you'd expect. They are not all skinny and ragged and desperate. Some of them have jobs, and good jobs, too. Their friends probably smoke a little weed and do a few lines of coke now and then. But if your drug of choice happens to be heroin or crack, you'll struggle to get hold of it if you move in nice, middle-class circles. So you have to venture down into the sewers. Most times, I guess, you take your fix, drift off and stumble home when you come round. Mr Shiny Shoes just never came round.

DRUNK

Most people like a drink. Most of them occasionally have a bit too much to drink.

Some people take it a lot further than that.

Every Friday night, they get dressed up and head into town. They start drinking at about 6pm, and they don't stop until 2am, or 3am, or 4am. They stick glasses in people's faces in nightclubs and get into fights in chip shops. They put their fists through shop windows and urinate in doorways. They have sex with strangers in alleyways and vomit in the gutter. They brawl with the police. They fall over and hit their heads. They walk out into the road and get hit by cars. They collapse unconscious, dehydrated, poisoned with the sheer amount of drink they've taken.

They do the same on Saturday night. Increasingly, they do it on any night of the week.

All those broken noses, smashed jaws, lacerated tendons, glassings and booze-induced head injuries end up in our hands. And they're just the immediate problems: the hidden effects of the alcohol in which our country is drowning will catch up with us in the years to come, I can assure you of that.

The practical effect of all this is felt by you, even if you're not out kicking in phone boxes or punching people: the taxpayer funds the emergency services, after all. I don't know exactly how many of the calls I attend are drink-related, but it runs into hundreds each year. Certainly, on a typical Thursday, Friday, Saturday and sometimes Sunday night, most of my calls will be alcohol-related; 'ETOH', we call them. The acronym refers to Ethyl Alcohol (chemical formula $CH3CH2OH$), which is grain alcohol and so generally used to describe any relative alcoholic condition. It's an inaccurate term, but well suited when we want to write 'drunk' or 'affected by alcohol', or are tempted to use other, less academic-sounding terms.

It's worst of all among the young and dangerous. They believe that alcohol enhances their sex appeal. I can tell you that the sight of a swearing, vomiting woman - I've seen a few, and I don't care if she's a model in a miniskirt - has never been attractive to me. Likewise few sober girls get turned on by a guy staggering around, out of his tree.

They spend hundreds of pounds a week on booze and a few of them inevitably end up with a needle in their arm and a bag hanging from it. For some, just as ASBOs have become symbols of street credibility, IV lines and fluid are becoming the hallmark of a perfect evening of social interaction.

It doesn't look like getting any better in the near future, either. Drinking has almost become a national pastime for our kids. According to research, more than 80% of 11-16 year olds have tried booze, even if that was only to have a few sips. Most of them will grow up believing that it's a social necessity. In my own family, my teetotal older brother was the only one to abstain completely from drinking. I still remember the looks he got when I took him to a pub with my mates one time and he ordered a pint of milk. It's almost a crime *not* to drink in modern Britain.

Speaking of crime, the Home Office says alcohol is responsible for almost half of the violence that scars this country every weekend and, increasingly, every day. It certainly sucks up a good chunk of NHS resources. And every time someone calls an ambulance or the police because of an alcohol-related incident, you - the taxpayer - are forking out. The Government thought the problem would ease with the introduction of 24-hour drinking. The great minds of Westminster thought a 'cafe culture' would develop and people would drink in moderation because there was no need to rush.

You may as well introduce 24-hour fast food restaurants and say fat people will eat less.

We are being swamped, and the prospect for the future care and deliverance of alcoholics and other problem drinkers is bleak. It will cost the taxpayer more each year if we allow the trend to go on. Assaults will increase, alcohol-related deaths will increase and the financial burden will spiral ever higher, affecting each and every one of us, teetotallers included. Unless there is a money tree orchard somewhere I don't know about.

Excuses for being so drunk that you cannot stand, or control your bladder or gag reflex, include 'I think my drink was spiked' and 'I only had three pints of lager and I've had much more than that in the past'. This misunderstanding of the nature of alcohol and its collision processes within our bodies leads to a very heavy NHS workload on a Friday and Saturday night.

A common call for me is to a *'collapsed female, possibly drunk'*. They usually are, and when I get on scene I am greeted with the same words.

'She's never been like this before.'

'Has she been drinking?' I'll ask as she vomits on my boots and flops around on the pavement.

'Yes, but not a lot.'

'What's 'not a lot' - a little, or some, or many?' I find sarcasm is missed by the drunken, so I can usually get away with it, watching my words flying over their heads and into the sunset (or sunrise, it's a 24-hour thing now, remember).

'Well, not a lot. She's only had three or four.'

This is normal. Nobody ever gives me the exact number of drinks that have been consumed, neither do they tell me what *kind* of alcohol and in what measure it has been taken. Anecdotally, it seems that women who are menstruating get drunk quicker. Research carried out by The University of Chicago disputes this, but I've lost count of the number of times I've treated collapsed, drunken females who have been on or are near to their period. It's almost become an instinctive question for me to ask them when I arrive on scene. This is definitely worth further study, I feel.

In men, it's usually down to a lack of food. Lining your stomach does work - food helps to absorb some of the alcohol before it reaches the gut (where it is quickly taken up by the bloodstream). In my experience, blokes are more likely to ignore this common sense approach, so they face a depletion of sugar as a result of their recent fast and then the alcohol inhibits the release of supplies from their liver. This causes hypoglycaemia and it can lead to collapse. In fact, as few as two drinks can cause a sudden drop in blood sugar.

BM. Blood glucose monitoring. We measure blood glucose levels in almost every patient we attend, and in drunks as a matter of routine. The test involves pricking the skin to obtain capillary blood which is then placed on a measuring strip and into a light-reflecting meter. The meter (a glucometer) measures the level of glucose in the blood. Normal levels are between 4 and 10mmol. A reading below 4mmol indicates hypoglycaemia. Anything above 10mmol is called hyperglycaemia but is not necessarily dangerous until the levels reach the high teens. (Mmol stands for millimoles per litre; a 'millimole' is 1/1000th of a mole and a mole is a molecular measurement.)

I went to the aid of a man who had become unresponsive after a heavy night of drinking. He was slumped against some railings next to a Kentucky Fried Chicken takeaway in the East End. His friends were gathered around him, unsure of what to do; they were about to lift him into a taxi when I showed up. It's just as well they didn't - when I examined him I found that his blood glucose level was seriously low. If he'd been left at home in his current state, he may have slipped into a coma before his body had time to recover and release much-needed glucose. That could have led to death.

Luckily, he was able to accept oral glucose when I gave it to him; Glucagon (which helps release stored glucose in the liver) would have been of little use, because the elimination of alcohol was keeping his liver busy and so the hormone wouldn't have been able to do its job.

Combining drugs - of any kind - with alcohol is just asking for trouble. I've treated plenty of individuals who have taken their prescription meds, including anti-depressants, with drink. Notwithstanding the high risk to their liver, the result is a collapsed and usually very depressed person.

I have seen two or three examples of extremely unusual behaviour as a result of mixing business with pleasure. I remember one woman who was out on a works do with her colleagues. She'd had far too much to drink and I was called to the pub to help her. When I got there, I found a middle-aged lady lying on a sofa in the bar, thrashing around and screaming at the top of her voice for absolutely no reason. Every time I tried to speak to her I was met with a hateful glare and a mute response. I had to lean forward to grab her several times to stop her falling onto the hard floor, and was rewarded with a series of blows for my trouble. At one point, she stuck a finger in my eye, leaving me unable to focus for a while as my eye watered in protest. She relented only when the room was cleared of her work associates. Suddenly, she became a cooperative human being - only minutes before she had been a banshee. What's *that* all about? I never found out.

Drunks on buses have become familiar calls for me. I can guarantee that on every weekend shift I will find myself at some point boarding a bus, shouting at a sleeping figure and trying to wake it up in order to get it off the bus. (Bus drivers aren't allowed to do this apparently, they have to call an ambulance. They tend to use words like 'unconscious' or 'dead' to get the emergency response they need.)

I climbed aboard a No72 which had stopped on a high street after I had been summoned to an *'unconscious male on bus'* - that's the usual modus operandi for a sleeping drunk. The driver stood outside and pointed at the stairs.

'He's up there,' he said, his finger indicating the way. As if there was any other way to get to the top deck.

'Did you try to wake him?' I asked.

'Yes.'

'How?'

'I stood at the front and threw a shoe at him.'

I looked down at the bus driver's feet. Both his shoes were in place.

'What shoe?' I asked.

'His'.

Let's get this straight. He'd gone right up to this sleeping drunk, pulled off one of his shoes and lobbed it at him (smacking him on the head) in order to get his attention. And when that hadn't worked, he had dialled 999.

I went upstairs and saw the one-shoed man slumped across the back seat. He was big and he smelled bad. That might have been because his shoe was off and his sock was unhealthy. I shook him and shouted for him to wake up.

'Whaa!' he shouted back. He had a thick Russian or Polish accent. The most interesting change in recent times, for me, has been the massive shift in the nationality of drunks we deal with. We Scots have (had?) a reputation as boozers. It was never seen as a slur on the nation, just a broadly-brushed fact (though don't call us tight-fisted). Now East Europeans are showing up in ever-increasing numbers on the streets of the capital, and they're often off their faces. I mean, some of them have a real and incurable problem with drink. Of all the 'unconscious on a bus' or 'collapsed, unknown cause' calls

I've attended in the past year where the patient has been smashed, I would have to say that more than 70% of them have been Russian, Polish or Lithuanian. Remember, this is my own personal statistic; other ambulance service personnel may tell a different story.

'Time to get off. You are asleep on the bus,' I told him, with a friendly smile.

'Uh?'

'You need to leave the bus, now. Do you need an ambulance?' I think it's best to cover all the bases, just in case, although I hoped he'd say no.

'No,' he said

'Then you have to leave the bus. I'll walk you off, OK?'

'OK. I go,' he said. Then he glanced down to his feet and up at me again. He looked confused and more than a little upset.

'Where is shoe?' his angry, pink face demanded.

* * * * *

Another serious side-effect of alcohol consumption is the loss of body heat. It may make you feel warmer, but actually it lowers your core body temperature. If you get slaughtered and fall asleep outside you are at risk of hypothermia and death. Even in London, wearing nothing but a thin shirt and a pair of jeans is definitely asking for trouble, particularly if you're going to end up kipping on the pavement.

On a cold November night during a weekend FRU shift, I was asked to check on the status of a man *'lying in the street'*. When I read these words I am pretty sure I'm going to find a sleeping drunk, especially if I'm reading them on a weekend night.

I arrived to find a young man, lying on his back and out for the count, in a side street off The Strand. This part of town is usually busy up until the wee small hours, but it was now 4.30am and there wasn't a soul around - not at this end anyway. Whoever had called the ambulance had taken to his heels shortly afterwards - obviously too busy to stop and actually *do* anything.

I went up to the guy and prodded him a few times, but he didn't respond. He just lay there, arms folded, oblivious and unconscious. He was dressed in a cotton T-shirt and a pair of jeans. He had no head wear and nothing to protect his hands from the cold, except his pockets or his arm-pits and he wasn't using either at the moment.

I tried again, this time a little more energetically, but he remained resolutely unresponsive. Effectively, he was in a mini-coma. He was muscular and tall, and since he was a dead weight I knew I'd struggle to move him should I have to.

I ran my usual checks, but my main concern was with his temperature. His skin felt like ice but he wasn't shivering. Shivering occurs when the body attempts to create heat from muscular activity. It does this automatically when your core temperature drops by one or two degrees - your normal average body core temperature being around 37°C. The shivering mechanism becomes more violent as the temperature drops a further one or two degrees. After that, as heat continues to be lost, shivering stops - usually at around 32°C.

I covered him with foil and blankets and tried to take his temperature. The equipment we use takes measurements from the ear, but for a more accurate reading it should be taken rectally - luckily for you (and us), that is always done at hospital. Unfortunately, my thermometer wouldn't read properly. We'd both have to wait until an ambulance arrived to take him away.

In conscious people, as their body temperature falls, they exhibit strange behaviour. One key indicator is attempting to squeeze into the smallest spaces possible, like cupboards, in a vain and semi-lucid attempt to find warmth. This is known as 'terminal burrowing' and is often the last thing they do before they die. In an unconscious drunk, though, there is no way of knowing just how far down the line they are and how much the cold has affected their brain and other organs without an accurate core temperature.

During the journey he began to wake up, and by the time we arrived at A&E he was looking around, though he still wasn't fully conscious. His temperature was checked accurately and found to be 31.2°C. It took hours of passive re-warming to recover him fully and the next time I saw him, sitting up in bed chatting to a nurse about his adventures, I was just about to go home. It's entirely possible that, had he been left unnoticed, he would have died. Seriously, it's only a matter of time before I come across a young corpse, lying in the street in trendy clothes with a drunken smile on its face.

An American tourist summed it up for me as I was kneeling over a vomit-streaked girl in Whitehall a while back. 'Jeez,' he said. 'You have a lot of drunk people in the UK, don't you?'

We do, and it's not just bad for the drunks, or for tourism. It's also bad for the NHS - it's costly, of course, but it's killing morale. Not many of us joined this profession desperate to wade through as much drink, vomit and stupidity as we could. Most of us are here to care for people who really need it, not selfish self-harmers who go out of their way to blitz the system with their lifestyle problems.

My colleagues and I stand in the wasteland of other people's lives and watch as they destroy themselves in a bottle.

OLD

We don't take care of our elderly in this country. Many people live in the most appalling conditions - either at home, or while being abused and ignored in the less reputable 'care homes' - and very little is done about it. Apart from the odd *Panorama*-type programme to highlight the atrocities faced by our elder generation, not much is even said, publicly.

In 2003, the then Health Minister John Hutton stated that draft national rules on improving care standards in both the public and private sector would make 'horror stories of badly-run homes a thing of the past'. In my profession, I have seen and continue to see too many examples of neglect and abuse to believe his rules are working. In fact, a more recent report, published by the Joint Committee on Human Rights, said it was 'shameful' that a fifth of care homes in the UK were failing to meet minimum standards. Rhetoric changes nothing in the real world; no doubt our politicians and their parents will be well looked after, though.

Two calls I attended stick in my memory. Both of them were to nursing homes, and each involved a bed-ridden female who was on her last breath of life. On one of these calls, there was no proper hand-over, no medical care had been given, or had been attempted, and the patient smelled as if she had been lying in her own urine for days. The curtains had been drawn around her bed and she was left like this, as if she didn't exist, until we arrived and took her to hospital. She died later that day.

Another lady I went to when I was on lates had been left for hours with breathing problems before staff ventured to call an ambulance. Their excuse was that they didn't know she was having problems until they noticed her colour had changed (she was virtually blue by the time I saw her). My colleague had to intubate her in the back of the ambulance, and we made every attempt to recover her, but she, too, died in hospital after our fruitless resuscitation attempt.

We put in an official complaint but I don't think anything ever came of it. The old woman probably had no relatives to complain on her behalf.

> **LATES. These shifts start from lunchtime onward. Starting at 3pm has the benefit of allowing you to take your time getting ready for work. Unfortunately, you are jumping right into the middle of the day and will probably get called out the minute your feet touch the station floor.**

It's not just in some privately-run homes that our elderly are being abused. Researchers from the King's Institute of Gerontology in London spent two years collecting data on the problem and uncovered a horrifying figure of more than 700,000 cases, many of which occurred in the person's own home. The attitude of the 'carer' towards the person being cared for often deteriorated from simply being dismissive or ignoring the person's needs, to ever-increasing levels of abuse, including physical harm.

I was called to a house where an old man lived alone. He had chest pains and some difficulty breathing. I was working alone on the FRU, so I couldn't take the gentleman to hospital until an ambulance arrived. He was in his bedroom and I was led to him by a young 'carer', hired by the local authority to attend to the man's needs on a regular basis. She left me with him and wandered off without referring to me (or him) again.

I treated the man with oxygen for his breathing problem and I explained that he would have to wait for an ambulance. He became panicky and claimed that if he left the house, the carer would 'do things'. I didn't know whether his mild dementia was talking or he was being sincere, but he looked genuinely frightened and he went on to claim she was abusing him. I couldn't do anything to help because I had no proof. All I could do was record his claim on a form and submit it to my bosses. I had to leave him with the ambulance crew, but I could still hear him refusing to leave his home while she was still there.

Many of our elderly live in conditions that defy belief. I visit many houses where the access is blocked by rubbish and decades of 'collecting'. Useless items and boxes containing spare parts fill every room. I'll often find the patient behind, among or underneath these mountains of junk. Such situations increase the vulnerability of these people because they are unable to move around safely and can trip and fall at any time, often becoming lost in their household debris. The search for an injured old person can take a long time, especially when they're behind locked doors.

Add to this that they often live in conditions of poor hygiene and it can be extremely depressing. I've treated many elderly people who have been sitting there, covered in their own excrement. You don't need visual clues when you walk into a house like that; all you need is a rudimentary sense of smell.

* * * * *

One of the most vulnerable old ladies I ever came across refused to go to hospital and was left at home to her fate. My crewmate and I had been called to a house in north London to investigate a possible collapse. There was no reply from the front door, no matter how hard we banged on it, so we went around to the back. The police joined us and we peered into the sitting room through the patio doors.

There was an elderly lady slumped in a chair. She looked unconscious but when we rapped on the window, she looked up. We called in for her to come to the door but she motioned that she couldn't move. We tried to get in through the double glass doors but they wouldn't budge, so we ventured back round to the front.

The police officer tested the door to gauge how much of a kick it would need, but it was a shoddy, weak affair and as soon as he leant on it there was a creak and it gave way. No security. Anyone could have shouldered it in with little effort. Once inside, we went straight through to check on our patient. She was sitting in her armchair and looked terribly pale. She told us that she didn't need an ambulance and that she wanted to be left alone. She allowed a cursory examination and my crewmate found several bruises, caused by falling. She had damaged her hip (more than likely fractured it) and had soiled herself so badly that her dress stuck to the sofa. It looked like she had been in this position for days. Her bed was nearby, and she hardly left the room - her meals were delivered. The rest of her house, which was a fairly substantial four or five bedroom place worth a lot of money in the right hands, was falling into neglect. I stood looking at her, thinking how easily she could be robbed or worse while she slept. She was very vulnerable.

We asked her to prove that she could fend for herself and didn't need to go to hospital. 'Can you stand up and take a few steps?' I said. This was a risky strategy because if her hip was broken this could increase her pain and suffering. Reluctantly, she agreed, and stood on shaking legs. She tried to move, but she was completely unable to take a step and, as her pain increased, she collapsed back into the chair. She was injured and needed proper care, but she steadfastly refused.

'I want you to leave me alone,' she said. 'Just go away.'

We persuaded her that she wouldn't be forced to do anything, and that we just wanted to stay until we'd helped her. Meanwhile, we called her GP. He arrived after an hour or so and started trying to convince her she needed to go to hospital. But despite his best efforts, she wouldn't budge. As I looked at her face, wrinkled with age and pain, I realised that we were witnessing her fear; she was afraid that if she left she would never return. I understood that. She had probably lived here for 50 years, and the unknown was terrifying. I felt hopelessly inadequate.

I chatted with the police officer about removing her against her will, but she obviously had mental capacity: that meant she had the right to decide for herself what she did, and we'd be breaking the law if we tried to force her out. The paradox, of course, was that - objectively - the best thing for her was pain relief and medical attention.

We found her phone book and some family members were listed. Calls were made, but all efforts to get any of them down to help failed. None of them wanted to come. They didn't seem to care. I wondered why.

In the end, we left her with her GP but it looked like she was going to stay put. We were out of the loop now. It's an awful admission, and it felt like failure at the time. But I had envisaged her screaming and thrashing on the trolley bed as she was taken from the house and I imagined the faces of the hospital staff when we arrived with our stubborn patient. That wasn't a realistic way to treat anyone, so it didn't happen. I doubt she survived the night alone in that house, and if she did I very much doubt she lasted the week.

On a few calls, the result of a lack of care for the elderly is more subtle.

I was asked to go and assess a 93-year-old lady whose GP had requested a trip to hospital for an x-ray on her arm. When I got to the house and went in, the old lady's carer (and friend) took me to her and described what had happened. She'd bent over a few days earlier to pick up her post and had stumbled - something that's not at all uncommon in old folks. She'd fallen onto her arm, fracturing the humerus in the process. The humerus is a fairly big bone and a fracture to it can lead to serious complications. I consider it a potential emergency, especially in the elderly.

Nevertheless, she had been taken to hospital, examined and given a very simple, semi-rigid splint - the type of splint that is not sufficient to keep a bone absolutely still. She was sent home with some pain killers, and that was that. A day or so later, she had developed an uncomfortable swelling at her elbow below the site of the fracture. She'd asked her carer to remove the splint because the pain was increasing. This was done and it was never put back on. The carer called the specialist who had operated on this lady's shoulder previously and asked for advice about this new situation. She was told that as long as the old lady remained still and did not move much, the arm would get better on its own. It didn't; it got much worse.

When I examined her, I found a definite distortion of the shape of her mid-shaft humerus and saw that the swelling was a large and painful-looking haematoma. A haematoma forms when blood leaks into the tissues under intact skin; the fracture had moved and was now leaking blood, and possibly bone marrow, into her tissues - all of which was gathering in a large pool in her elbow. She had been sleeping on it, walking around with it and trying to live with it for four days.

I called an ambulance for her and made sure she got to hospital before the limb became too damaged to save.

When I took her blood pressure, I had to use a tiny child's cuff because she was so small and frail. 'Can you manage all right?' she asked me, as I adjusted it. It reminded me of the last time an old lady had shown concern for me. I'd been treating her for a suspected heart attack. I hadn't been doing the job long and I must have looked more nervous than she was.

ACTS OF VIOLENCE

As I've said, in the ambulance service we are exposed to violence on a regular basis. Mostly, it's directed towards someone else but, occasionally, it's aimed at us. I've been kicked, bitten and threatened whilst attending to the medical needs of patients, and in most cases alcohol was to blame for the aggressive behaviour. (Well, the aggressor was to blame, but the alcohol was a factor.) Sometimes we get assaulted simply because we represent something the patient doesn't like; uniforms, authority, the system. I don't know. Maybe it's the colour green... who can say?

It had been quiet on this particular day, and then Jack, a regular caller, called had rung in from the West End. I tracked him down to an alley in Chinatown. He'd called for chest pains again, though he never has them. He's very well-known and has a notorious history of exploiting the ambulance service. He's even gone as far as to fake his own stabbing to get the attention of all three services (I have no idea why the fire service turned up on that call).

On this particular night, I was working alone on the FRU and, since I knew Jack from many of his previous calls, I felt I could deal with him on my own. He has a violent streak, but he'd never been openly aggressive to me, so I didn't feel particularly worried. I was, however, determined to call his bluff and avoid wasting yet another ambulance on him.

His pattern of behaviour is always the same. He gets a member of the public to call 999, either by faking an illness or an injury, or simply by lying down and not moving for long enough to catch someone's attention. When the ambulance arrives he'll size up the crew; if they're new and they don't know him, he'll put on an Oscar-winning act of pain and suffering until he is taken to hospital. He was so good at this the first time I encountered him that I gave him IV pain relief.

> **QUIET. Actors never use the word 'Macbeth'. We never use the word quiet, at least not while we're on duty. If we do, a barrage of calls will suddenly come in for no logical reason whatsoever.**

Once at hospital, he will demand food and immediate attention. If he doesn't get what he wants, he trashes his cubicle, threatens and insults the nursing staff, and then storms out. He has done this in at least three different hospitals in Central London. You may think he has 'problems'. Yeah, right. He has called ambulances out as many as times five times in one day. Next time you need one urgently, remember that.

So, here I was standing in this alleyway telling him that he was not going to hospital this time because he was drunk and nothing else was wrong with him. He wasn't happy with me at all.

'You've got to take me to hospital, it's my right,' he said.

'No, I don't, Jack,' I said. 'You abuse your rights.'

'I'll call another ambulance when you go,' he said.

'No you won't, because I've told Control that you would probably do that.'

'F**k off then.'

He made as though to shuffle off, but suddenly turned and rounded on me, shouting in my face. I could smell the booze on his breath, and my face was flecked with his spit. I was nervous: he has convictions for assault and, so the story goes, did time for murder a long while back. 'I'm gonna call you lot every hour of the day,' he shouted. 'I'm gonna make sure you f**king ambulance people get what's coming to you.'

Then he spat at me.

I backed off a little and as I did so he ran to a wall and picked up a bottle. He headed back towards me, brandishing it like a club. Either he was going to smash it over my head, or it was all front; I stood my ground. It wasn't bravery; I had nowhere else to go, to be honest.

'Put the bottle down!' I shouted, loud enough to attract the attention of pedestrians on the road outside the alley. 'Don't be stupid.'

He hesitated.

'Put it down!' I said again, as firmly as I could.

This time, only feet away from me, he relented, choosing to swear some more at me instead. It was a close call, and it made me much more wary of him whenever I saw him again, but he never gave me any more grief afterwards. He still calls ambulances, and I suspect he is behind a lot of hoax calls received from his 'patch'.

You're probably wondering why we don't 'do something' about Jack. Well, I've called the cops to him a few times, and they come and pour his drink down the drain and get him to move on. They don't bother arresting him and I can understand that - all he'd get is a week in the cells and it's not worth the hours of paperwork to put him there. But lately, he's been calling in and asking for all three emergency services and then hanging up. So I race round to an empty phone box, and by the time I get there he's called in again from somewhere else. We end up playing a game of 999 hopscotch with him around Soho. We know it's him, but proving it is hard.

So why don't we just refuse to go? Well, the bosses are scared that someone is going to drop dead after we have told them that we are not coming out. Personally, I think that would be a bonus - it's only a matter of time before he costs someone else *their* life, after all. I went to one of his hoax calls recently. I got to the call box; he wasn't there so I greened up. Immediately, up popped a call that had been waiting for 10 minutes. It was to a four-year-old girl, DIB, on the other side of town. Thank God the kid wasn't serious, but if she had been, and she'd died, Jack would have been directly to blame. And there's not a damn thing that we could have done about it.

* * * * *

Domestic disputes often spill into real violence when drink is involved, and I have treated a number of women who have been the victims of their partner's fury or drunken aggression. Some of the injuries I have treated have been serious. The Home Office says domestic violence accounts for 16% of all violent crime in England & Wales and claims the lives of more than 100 women a year (and 30 men). The cost is enormous - more than £23 billion a year.

Women who receive grievous injuries still try to defend their aggressor (it's usually their husband or partner), though nowadays the police can prosecute without the need for the victim to press charges.

We received a call to a young woman at a block of flats in the dead of night. She had allegedly been assaulted and the police were not yet on scene. We went in, blissfully unaware of what had happened. The flat was eerily quiet and there was broken glass around the hall.

THE POLICE. Our best friends, bar none (though closely followed by the men and women of the London Fire Brigade). The Met police and BTP are pretty much always on our side, because they see what we are up against every single day (and night). They're usually on scene, and they watch our backs and keep us safe. Like the LFB, they also make excellent drip stands. God bless you all.

I suddenly became more cautious and shouted into the front room.

'Hello? Ambulance.'

There was a sobbing reply from inside the room - it was the young woman we had come to help.

'I'm in here,' she said.

We went into the room and she was sitting on a chair, dressed in her night clothes and shakily smoking a cigarette. Her face was smeared with old and current tears and she had minor cuts to her neck and arms. As I examined her, she told us what had happened.

'I had an argument with my boyfriend and he started punching and kicking me,' she explained. 'Then he went into the kitchen while I was on the floor and he brought one of the knives out.' She looked terrified. 'I thought he was going to kill me, I really did.'

She started to cry again and we settled her down. We were all a little on edge. I walked into the kitchen and there, on the table, was a large carving knife. The sight of it sent a shiver down my spine.

When I returned to the front room, my crewmate was chatting to the young woman, who was busily dialling a number on her mobile phone. She looked up at us both and said that she didn't want her boyfriend to get into trouble.

'I'm going to ask him to come back so we can sort this out between us,' she said.

My jaw probably dropped but I don't remember for sure. 'No,' I said (I may have shouted). 'You can't bring him back here.'

'Why not?'

'He's dangerous and he'll put us at risk.'

'No, he won't. He's harmless really. He'll be sorry for what he did now.'

I couldn't believe my ears, but I have seen this so many times that I should have anticipated it. She'll have gone through it all again and again in the past; it's become part of her life; but I sure as hell didn't want to be introduced to her violently passive boyfriend.

The police arrived before she could get through. They began to interview her. She told them what she had told us, insisting that she didn't want to press charges or go to hospital. She had received her care and attention, and now all she wanted was to be left alone so that she could reunite herself with her aggressive other half. True love.

Some families have their own way of settling scores and they wait for opportune moments, when alcohol is flowing freely, to do just that. A call to a 'fight at party' turned out to be a serious assault at a wedding reception being held by a travelling family. We pulled up outside the venue and found police on scene and a lot of menacing faces hanging about. We weren't a welcome sight. In fact, I got the distinct impression that nothing with blue lights was welcome.

The injured man had been attacked in what the papers would probably call 'a drink-fuelled frenzy'. He had nasty facial injuries, the worst of which was to his ear; it had been bitten off, leaving only a ragged pulp of bloody flesh on the side of his head. There was considerable bleeding and that had to be controlled first.

As he was treated, the man stared straight ahead with his wife and family looking on. I think his mind was busy with thoughts of revenge, rather than the serious nature of the wound, and he was also very pale and sweaty, so we moved him onto the trolley bed to keep his blood pressure up. Ideally, we needed to find the missing ear, so I asked around and eventually was pointed in the direction of where the 'party' had been taking place. I found myself standing in a large hall which looked, literally, like a bomb had gone off in it; they had trashed the place, either as a consequence of having a good time or during the fight (there had been a number of people involved).

A venue manager was standing there, looking slightly dazed.

'I don't suppose you've seen an ear lying about, mate?' I said.

He just pointed to a large bin. I looked into the bin and started rummaging around among the half-eaten sausage rolls and pizza crusts. In the end, I had to admit defeat: the guy needed to go to hospital, the ear was proving elusive and even if I did find it the chances of it being in pristine nick had diminished to almost zero considering where it had been stored. So I went back empty-handed and we took the man to hospital for some urgently needed repair. I don't know if he was a qualifying case for plastic surgery, but I doubt it; the ear was most likely stitched up and left to heal over into a ragged stump. He'd have a nice battle scar to show off to his friends and family. Personally, I'd rather have an ear.

Knives are never far from a modern-day fight, and they have produced some of the worst wounds I've treated. Many of the patients were innocent bystanders; they were just in the wrong place at the wrong time when 'it all kicked off'. One or two of them, with relatively minor nicks, didn't even know they had been stabbed until the blood was pointed out; others never stood a chance.

On a horrible, rainy night, my crewmate and I were called to a stabbing at an address in north London. We arrived on scene to see another crew bringing a patient out of the small terraced house on a trolley bed. They were resuscitating, and there was a lot of blood around. A lot. We joined them in their vehicle and I saw the extent of the injuries immediately. Lying on the bed was a young woman, probably in her early twenties. She had been stabbed a number of times and I could see at least two wounds, both in her chest. Her blood, red and sticky and metallic-smelling, was washing around the ambulance floor now.

I started working on her airway and breathing whilst CPR continued. The HEMS team arrived within a few minutes and I intubated her as they set about organising themselves with the crew. I saw a flash in my peripheral vision and thought nothing of it, but when I asked for a stethoscope so that I could check that my tube had entered the correct pipe and the lungs were filling with air, the doctor said, 'Why don't you just have a look?'

The patient's chest was gaping open. The flash had come from the doctor's cutting instruments - he had performed a thoracotomy (like the one nearly performed on the Scottish one-under discussed earlier) so that he could get to the heart directly and massage it. There was no need for me to check her lungs with a stethoscope, I could see them rising and falling.

With the amount of blood she had lost, she needed fluids. But her veins had collapsed, making IV access impossible, so I carried out an intraosseous access (the first time I'd performed this procedure, actually). This involves using a thick and pretty nasty-looking needle to cut through the bone and into the marrow cavity so that fluids can be given where there is no venous access. I tried several times, once in each shin bone (one of which was successful) and once in the pelvis, which also worked. Unfortunately for the woman, no amount of fluid was going to help her and she was pronounced dead in the ambulance.

This was one of the nastiest, bloodiest assaults I have dealt with to date, and if I never see a worse one I'll be happy. The woman's husband had stabbed her several times in the chest and back, and then ran off as the police were arriving, or so the story went. I don't think he got far.

That same night, at another location, I was attending a young man who had gone home bleeding from a wound in his chest. He had told his family that he had been 'punched', but his condition had deteriorated so much that they had called an ambulance. His breathing wasn't right and he was as pale as a ghost. Externally, the wound looked small and insignificant, but I had no idea how deep it was. As I examined him, he started going into shock, so I had to assume he had lost more blood than we could see. We wasted no time getting him to hospital.

The sad truth is, my colleagues and I could fill a book with the random assaults we come across.

A call to a petrol station in the City one Saturday night for a 'collapsed male' turned out to be a little more complicated. I found him lying on the floor of the little shop. He had come in, staggered to the counter and collapsed. He was conscious but very frightened looking.

'What's happened?' I asked

'I've been beaten up by four men for no reason,' he said.

I looked at his arms, which were bruised and bleeding, and then I realised his wounds were not the result of a simple beating. He had long, deep cuts to his arms and a few oval punctures to his neck and face.

'Did you see a weapon when they beat you up?'

'No, I don't think so. Why?'

'I think you've been stabbed,' I said.

I went on to tell him that his wounds were not dangerous, but there was no doubt in my mind that the intentions of his assailants were deadly. They had tried to stab his neck and throat, narrowly missing his carotid artery and jugular vein. His arm wounds were probably defensive and, I thought, had quite likely saved his life.

'S**t,' he said. 'Serious?'

I called the police and requested an ambulance for him.

Another hapless victim of this kind of violence was walking down the street minding his own business when he was accosted for his mobile phone. He refused to give it up and was rewarded with a blade to his eye. The knife penetrated just underneath the eyeball and pierced it from beneath. Whether he will recover his sight or not will be down to the skill of the doctors and a lot of luck.

A similar call had me attending a young man who had been stabbed. He'd been approached and stabbed in the leg before the muggers demanded his phone. He had handed it over, and wasn't resisting, but the assailants had then tried to stab him again - this time in the chest. He'd stopped the knife with his hand, which was now sliced open. I was shocked at the ferocity of his attackers. They had what they wanted but they still tried to kill him. I didn't see the point, unless the point isn't just to gain the prize but a reputation too.

The other weapon of choice for our evil youth is guns. The Home Office report on gun crime in the UK shows a steady rise in shootings to almost 4,000 in 2006. The number of fatalities associated with these crimes has remained steady, however, with the number of serious or slightly-injured victims increasing. Whether this reflects the amateur nature of the shooter, who generally belongs to a gang and has no real weapons training, or a deliberate culture of shooting for punishment and as a means of terror, I don't know, but the threat is clearly real and the incidence is on the rise.

On every shooting I have attended, the police were required to place armed officers at the entrance and exit to the Resus room in case of reprisal. Shooters don't want their victims to survive and become witnesses.

In London, most of these crimes involve young black men. Sometimes they are gang members, sometimes they are drug dealers, sometimes they are just innocent people who found themselves in the way of a bullet. For all of us in the ambulance service, they are just kids and, sometimes, they are dead kids.

I remember working in a quieter part of London, where gun crime is not so much of a problem, when an ambulance crew brought in a 17-year-old lad who had just been gunned down in the street. He was being resuscitated aggressively as they brought him out of the vehicle and blood was pumping out of three wounds in his chest. There wasn't a chance in hell as far as I could see, and the Resus team agreed soon afterwards.

His family arrived shortly after he was pronounced dead, and the noise of their understandable grief drowned out all of the usual hospital sounds around me. It erupted suddenly, and continued for a long time afterwards. I got the distinct impression that they were good people, and that their son had been another innocent statistic, ripped from them suddenly, terribly. I wondered what could ever console them, and I realised that nothing could or would. Except perhaps time.

BRINGING THEM BACK

Resuscitation carries with it the high risk of failure. A few years ago, your chances of survival - even with a bunch of us working on you - were minimal at best. Only around 5% of people would survive a full-blown resuscitation with defibrillation. Now, though, the probability of survival is much better, thanks chiefly to the new CPR guidelines, introduced in 2006. We concentrate more on the compressions (that's when you push down on the person's chest), the drugs and the shock side of things than we do with airway and breathing (so mouth-to-mouth is often left until later). The changes came after research suggested concentrating on these areas would bear more fruit, and I have to say that it does. I've witnessed the near-miraculous results of this new approach a few times now.

I have contributed to the successful resuscitation of at least five patients in recent years. In all, they equate to a third of my 'suspended' calls during that time. I am tremendously proud of this, as I'm sure my colleagues are with their own successes: that means five mums, dads, brothers or sisters are back home, instead of in the ground. But although we're getting better, death will always have the upper hand. We still have to cope with the probability, if not the near-inevitability, of fatality when we go to these calls. Yes, I've saved five, but that still means two thirds of my patients *didn't* make it.

Before the new guidelines were introduced, a colleague and I were on a fairly routine night shift and received a call to a collapsed female. As we approached the scene, the call was upgraded to a 'suspended'. We looked at each other; this was my colleague's first suspended call as a paramedic, and it would be a test of her skills and knowledge.

There was an EMT already on scene - he was on the FRU that day - and we walked into the house and found him resuscitating the patient. She was a large woman who was lying half in and half out of the world's smallest toilet. Her husband stood in the front room watching as his wife's life hung in the balance. We started to unpack our equipment, but the hallway was so small that it quickly became a chaotic mess, with drugs, intubation and infusion packs strewn all around. My colleague took charge of the situation and attempted to intubate the woman whilst I got on with preparing the drugs and gaining IV access. Her airway was so messy (she had vomited) that getting into the trachea was proving very difficult. The little hallway was very dimly lit and there was no room for manoeuvre. Everything had to be done in a crouching position. Even the EMT had to straddle the woman to get on with the chest compressions properly. Everyone was having difficulty with this one.

The intubation attempts failed again and again, so the patient was ventilated using basic techniques whilst the trolley bed was brought into the house. There was no change in her condition; she had been in asystole (that means she showed no electrical activity or heartbeat) for some time now, and it was looking hopeless.

We lifted her onto the trolley bed and got her into the ambulance. CPR continued all the way to hospital and, for a short time, in Resus. At one point we thought they had some cardiac activity again but as we left I heard the doctor 'call it' and pronounce her dead. My colleague was devastated. She had wanted a positive outcome, but that rarely happened in those days. I tried to reassure her. Going from 'green' to 'experienced' with cardiac arrest management is not easy and it doesn't happen overnight. We don't have the same kind of support that is often provided in hospital. In the ambulance service, a paramedic must learn to carry the responsibility for every mistake made until there are so few (or none at all) that he or she becomes confident. I'm not suggesting that patient outcome suffers as a consequence, because there is usually someone on scene with enough experience to ensure the job is going to plan, but the outcome for this kind of call is always uncertain, even now and even with years of good quality CPR under a belt.

The next call we received for cardiac arrest was during an early shift. We were sent less than two hundred metres to a 'woman, collapsed in street - now suspended'. *This time*, I thought, *we'll do better*.

We were first on scene. It was a quiet street of Victorian terraces. A small group of people was standing around a woman lying on the pavement. We cleared a way through to her and confirmed that she was in cardiac arrest. I was attending this time round, so I took charge of the resus while my crewmate fetched the equipment from the ambulance. CPR was quickly taken over by a FRU colleague who arrived within a few minutes. I intubated the patient and my crewmate gained IV access and gave the first drugs. A shock had been delivered because the woman was in ventricular fibrillation (VF). My feeling was that there was an outside chance of saving her.

VENTRICULAR FIBRILLATION, or 'VF'. A chaotic electrical state in which the heart muscle is contracting in a random, inefficient way. The pumping ability of the heart ceases when VF occurs and unless the condition is reversed within a few minutes, using an electrical charge - defibrillation, with the paddles applied to the chest - the heart will eventually stop working altogether and the patient will die.

A couple had stopped with their two small children to watch this spectacle and I had to shoo them away. I still don't understand why parents think this is good entertainment for their kids.

They walked away.

As soon as we were able to, we moved the woman from the pavement to the ambulance and I continued CPR en-route to hospital. After a shock was delivered, I got a pulse and I asked my crewmate to slow down. I checked for breathing, but there was nothing, then the pulse went again. This happened three times on the way; a pulse appeared for a few seconds and then went again. It was very frustrating. It's a crude metaphor, but to me it's like lighting a fire, when the kindling keeps catching momentarily and then going out again. All you want is for the damned thing to take hold. 'Stay with me,' I said. 'Come on.'

When we had transferred her, we'd taken with us a bag that she had been carrying and which she'd dropped on the ground. We checked the contents and found a Blockbuster DVD and a shopping list. She'd never made it to the shops, and now she never would: she was pronounced dead soon after arriving at hospital. I felt bitterly disappointed, but both my colleague and I knew that we had managed this one much better.

Messy resus jobs are all too common for us and they present challenges that can test your skills to the limit. I went through a busy period of trial and error before I finally understood my role and how to play it.

The last call I received on one of my Christmas shifts was to a 'man collapsed, not breathing'. This happened in a large shopping centre, and security had called an ambulance because they thought the man might be dead. They didn't bother to approach him or start resuscitation, however, and I got a call from Control informing me that he might not be suspended at all and that others had called to say he was simply drunk.

I got on scene and an ambulance arrived simultaneously. The crew had been given a completely different description of the call and I was the only one unloading equipment for the possibility of a suspended. 'Tell you what,' I said, doubts filling my mind. 'Why not bring in your FR2 (defibrillator)?' I was probably wrong, but there was no harm in being prepared.

As soon as we got into the main entrance of the shopping centre a man came running toward us, waving and shouting that we needed suction. We all looked at each other; clearly, this wasn't just a drunk. So we ran up the escalator and down a corridor and found a chap lying on the floor. He was being resuscitated by a solo motorcycle paramedic who had arrived minutes earlier and who had also been caught out by the vague call descriptions. Nevertheless, something was now being done for the patient.

When I got closer I noticed a lot of vomit on the floor. This is always a bad sign. If a suspended patient vomits the airway becomes badly compromised and the lungs will take in fluid, a situation made worse when ventilating as it all gets blasted further down the bronchial tree. We pulled the man over (he was a BIG guy) and a lot more vomit poured from his mouth and nose onto the floor. The bike paramedic had not been able to intubate the man because he was working alone and the airway was so full of fluid that nothing could be seen properly (intubating blind is a big risk, for the reasons I've explained).

So we worked on him: me, the solo, and the paramedic and the EMT from the ambulance. We used our drugs and we tried to intubate him properly. The tube simply wouldn't go where it was needed and we were stuck with basic airway management and a suction machine that couldn't cope. We could have 'stayed and played' longer to try and change the situation - maybe even stabilise him - but it was looking dire so we got him into a chair, wheeled him out of the place and into the ambulance. CPR continued all the way to hospital. He was handed over in Resus and I didn't stay long enough to see what the outcome was, but I had no illusions.

A suspended octogenarian won't have much of a chance. The call had come in as a 'faint, not breathing at all' strangely enough - if you've fainted, you're normally breathing, but I guess that's the kind of confusion that takes over when you are elderly and a loved one has suddenly dropped to the floor. (Personally, I hope that's how I go.)

I worked on him with a crew and another FRU responder and, I have to say, it was fruitless from the start. His heart had given up and there was no way on earth it was going to pump again. This was a hard-working man who had probably lived a full life. I don't think he would have appreciated any extra time if he had been given it - the quality of life after delayed CPR is usually very poor if you recover at all; the brain will have been starved of oxygen and significant damage will have occurred. Nevertheless, we spent half an hour trying our best and achieving nothing. The bravest person in the room was his brother, who had to bear the sights and sounds of our efforts, only to be told that there was nothing else we could do. We stopped when inevitability became reality and left him on a sofa, wrapped in a blanket with his eyes closed, waiting for the undertaker. He looked asleep and that was a nice way to leave him, I think.

An early morning call to a 55-year-old female with 'no heartbeat' was given as 'suspended' by Control. There was already a crew on scene but they always send a few of us to a job like this.

I arrived and pressed the entry button for the flats. A few seconds later I was buzzed in by a crying female. I entered the lift and when I got out I could hear her wailing from all the way down the corridor. Neighbours were flitting in and out of their own flats, wondering what was going on.

I was let into the flat by one of the crew, who guided me upstairs. The paramedic was downstairs with the crying woman, so I knew that nothing was being done for the patient. When I got to the bedroom, I saw that the lady lying on the floor had been dead for some time, probably since the night before - nothing *could* be done. I went downstairs and joined the crew, who were consoling the young woman, the deceased's daughter. She was completely beside herself with grief.

She had gone to wake her mum up this morning and had found her. She kept saying, over and over again, that her mother must have been crying out for her in the night but that she hadn't heard. 'I must have just slept through while she was dying,' she said, between sobs. I looked at the stiff, discoloured corpse; the mouth and eyes were wide open and this had given the woman the impression that her mother must have been crying out as she died. This isn't necessarily true. The last few breaths taken by a dying person are usually taken after consciousness has slipped away - they are the body's desperate responses to a drop in oxygen levels, and are essentially nervous reflexes. If the last muscular reflex leaves the mouth open, then it will seem as if the person has screamed.

I felt devastated for the daughter; her mum was only 51. I arranged for the police to attend (the daughter was too upset to remember their GP's details) and left the scene when they turned up a few minutes later. It was a sad way to start the shift.

On an early evening call I was asked to assist with a crew who were working on a suspended alcoholic. He was only 45 and had been found in bed at his hostel, vomiting blood as a result of a massive internal bleed (gastro-intestinal). This brought about a cardiac arrest in front of the key worker who was trying to help him. When I arrived the crew were busily working on him on the floor. It was a pretty awful sight: there was a good deal of blood around, and his airway was a mess. The paramedic was attempting to intubate and I could see it

118

wasn't an easy job for him, but he got the tube in and secured it while I set about gaining IV access and preparing the drugs that would be needed. There are some jobs you just look at once and decide there is little or no hope. This was one of those jobs.

Still, we frantically ventilated, compressed and drugged him until another crew arrived to help with the removal to hospital. I had been on scene for about ten minutes and there was absolutely no change in the man's condition. The prognosis was poor. We prepared to move him downstairs (he was a large man and the stairwell, as usual, was very narrow) and tidied up our equipment. I asked the key worker and another member of staff to help carry the bags as we moved the resus effort from upstairs to downstairs and then into the ambulance. The first crew on scene conveyed the man to hospital and I took the key worker in the car so that he could pass on next-of-kin details to the hospital staff.

In the Resus room, work continued and many more people got involved, but it was called by the doctor in charge and the man was pronounced dead. Forty minutes after he had arrested.

I went back to the flat with the key worker because I had forgotten one of my bags and the place looked like it had been raided. The detritus of our effort was everywhere and there was plenty of evidence of recent death; blood on the floor, a crimson pillow on the bed and a little trail of the stuff leading from the flat to the outside world. In the bathroom, the man had prepared his shaving kit for the next day, not knowing that he wouldn't live to see it. I always find those innocuous little scenes of seeming normality very poignant.

* * * * *

A few days later I took a call to a collapsed middle-aged woman outside the National Portrait Gallery in St Martin's Place.

119

It was Red 1, high priority, but the details were scant. I called in. 'Can you tell me whether this person is suspended or not?'

They came back and confirmed that it was a suspended - the lady was reportedly not breathing and had no heartbeat - so I put my foot down a bit more. We were there in a couple of minutes. She was a German tourist who had dropped down in the street in sudden cardiac arrest. It was daylight and very busy, but an FRU EMT was on scene and there were a few other helpful people around. I had a training team with me - this was their first ever resus - and while they couldn't really do very much, they could fetch and carry and help out here and there. The EMT had started CPR; as the first and only paramedic on scene I had to take charge.

'Right,' I said. 'Can everyone just stop what you're doing for a sec while I check her out?'

Her worried husband was leaning over, watching me, and a crowd was gathering around. Other people were basically walking through the scene, which was shocking - a woman was dying here. I got the trainee crew to disperse everyone and set about trying to cannulate her. I failed - I couldn't get the needle in properly - so I moved on to securing her airway by intubating her. Another ambulance crew showed up to help and as they parked up I looked over. Right next to me was a man apparently trying to cannulate her. He wasn't ambulance service, and I didn't recognise him; he was just a random bloke in shirt and trousers. I said, 'What are you doing?'

He was a Canadian. He said, 'I'm a doctor, I thought I'd help out.'

'No,' I said. 'Can you please get away from my patient? I don't want you touching her.'

I didn't know whether he was a doctor or not - people claim all sorts of things - but even if he was, this was my patient, I was responsible for her and I didn't want anyone else working on her except ambulance service people.

But he wasn't getting the message. In a petulant voice, he said, 'Do you want me to get a line into her or not?'

'No,' I replied. Apart from anything else, I could see that he wasn't that experienced at it; he was messing around with the vein, getting nowhere.

He didn't move.

'I insist,' I said. So reluctantly he sloped off.

There's a common misconception, brought about from movies like *Flatliners*, that we can restart a totally inert heart with a defibrillator. You can't shock them out of it, it's usually too late. However, this lady's heart was in ventricular fibrillation. A heart in VF is not dead, but it's not pumping - it's kind of wobbling. The defibrillator shocks it, stops it dead for a split second, and this - we hope - allows the brain to kick it off again, like restarting a stalled car. (In some circumstances, it can convert into something called VT, ventricular tachycardia, which is a fast rhythm; this is also not life-sustainable, and if it appears drugs are usually used to slow the heart and get a proper rhythm back.)

We gave the lady a shot of adrenaline and prepared to shock her. Inevitably, this involves cutting her clothes off. Everything, bra included. There are obviously issues here, particularly for women, and while this patient was completely unaware of what was going on, we still had to respect her. To save her modesty, I asked my trainee crew to fetch blankets from the ambulances and got the police and passers-by to hold them up around her as a screen. Meanwhile, others police shepherded nosey tourists away.

After the first shock her heart got a rhythm back. This was an excellent sign. Another movie fallacy is that people wake up and are almost back to normal immediately. They don't. The first, often the only, sign you see is electrical evidence that they are back.

She was still unconscious and on the edge of death. We carried on with her breathing and moved her into the ambulance. We needed to get her to the hospital quickly. Our job is to stabilise the patient at the scene; we try not to move them until there is something salvageable, or there is no hope.

In the back of the ambulance, she started gagging, which was amazing. It meant she was coming round and trying to breathe for herself, and the tube was catching in her throat. I had never seen that happen before. Of course, we are trained to extubate, but I'd never had to do it because it's normally something that happens some time after the patient reaches hospital. I had to remind myself of the process, and as I was mentally working through it she opened her eyes. I told her I was going to take the tube out and I could see from her eyes that she understood.

Once it was out, she began to mouth words and eventually found her voice, which was croaky and weak because her voice box had been damaged by the tube. Another first: I've brought someone back and I'm having something of a conversation with her. I couldn't quite take it in; I'd been giving cardiac drugs and shocks to her just a few minutes before. She had been to the edge of life and looked over the cliff, and we'd brought her back. A magical feeling.

And she survived. After being in VF for 20 or 25 minutes, which is pretty good going. The EMT had got there within three minutes, and we'd been a minute or so later. Someone else - maybe the Canadian doctor - had been working on her before that, with manual CPR. That person actually saved her life because it kept her in a condition that we could work with, but the drugs and the defibrillation made the difference.

I went back up to the intensive care unit two or three days later and met her husband. They had reintubated her and put her back to sleep because her heart was unstable; until it was stable, the doctors wouldn't let her breathe for herself. She had a long road ahead of her, but she was going to be fine in the long term.

Her husband was obviously grateful to us for what we'd done, but he was reserved in his gratitude, and this was typical: relatives of people you save don't tend to behave like they do on *Casualty*, there are no tears or hugs, they're pretty matter-of-fact. Patients, on the other hand, are effusive if you visit them afterwards.

The greatest sense of satisfaction I got out of it - apart from saving her life - was for my trainees. The fact that their first resus had ended so successfully was sure to inspire them, I felt.

Young people go into cardiac arrest too, but it's uncommon and when a call comes through for a young chest pain or suspended, unless there's trauma or a medical link, it's difficult to believe. Thus, when I received a call to a '27-year-old, suspended' I wasn't sure it was accurate. I looked again at the age and considered the odds. This was probably not as given but then I heard Control giving details of the job to a motorcycle paramedic and the word suspended was used again, so I adjusted my thinking. I stepped up a gear to get there as fast as I could; if this was genuine the patient had minutes to survive (it wasn't made clear whether CPR was already being carried out).

I found myself behind an ambulance that was on the way to the same job and armed police guided us into the area. I wondered if this was a shooting because there were armed cops everywhere. Later I realised they had nothing to do with it; the origin of the call was behind an embassy building. A few of the police officers were soon roped in to help us, though.

I went into the house and there were already a number of people dealing - two ambulance crews and one motorcycle paramedic. CPR was underway on a young woman lying on the floor and I offered my help. Most of the people on scene were paramedics, so every skill role was filled, except the drugs. I got my drugs pack out and selected what might be needed for the patient just as a shock was called and delivered. This single shock changed the young woman's fate - it brought her back. She began gasping and convulsing.

I suggested we load and go because there was nothing else we could do at this stage; she needed to be sorted out in hospital. I brought the trolley bed in with the help of an armed-to-the-teeth police officer and we lifted her onto it and wheeled her out to the ambulance. Absolutely no more time was wasted and I travelled with the convoy to the nearest Resus room, where she continued to struggle for survival.

The woman had just collapsed and gone into cardiac arrest without obvious cause. I still don't know to this day what happened to her. All I know is that she lived.

A 'routine' call for a 45-year-old male having an epileptic fit in a pub turned out to be nothing of the sort. The call details changed en-route to 'unconscious, ? cause' with information that read 'caller happy to manage patient'. That was encouraging; it meant the patient was probably conscious and not fitting any more.

'?' on our computer screens means 'query' or 'suspected'. The question mark symbol is in general use in medicine and is used when there is a suspicion of an injury or condition... or anything for that matter. Technically, the '?' is used when you cannot be sure - a closed fracture is a good example. Without an x-ray there is no way we can absolutely define the injury, even if we are sure we know what it is. An open fracture, where the bone is sticking out would not require a '?' - it's an obvious fracture.

When I arrived, there were people standing around outside the pub drinking their pints and chatting; another sign that I took to mean all was well inside. There was an ambulance already on scene, so I thought my role here was just to support or help them if they needed me. I went inside, pushing my way through more drinkers, and as they opened up I saw a crew on the floor working on a suspended patient. He had gone into cardiac arrest almost as soon as they had arrived. They had already delivered one shock and the paramedic was intubating him and his crewmate was compressing the man's chest.

I looked around and realised the audience of punters were obstructing the exit. Some of them were even attempting to buy more booze as the resus took place below them near the bar.

That moment on the telly when the woman with the paddles shouts 'Clear!' is for a reason: that's a major electric shock you're delivering to the patient, and anyone touching the patient will get it, too. 'Can we just clear this area,' I shouted. 'Move away please.' It was for their own safety, but the lack of respect some of them showed for us and the dying man on the floor was shocking. It took me a while to get them, grudgingly, to give us some space.

The crew had done a stunning job and before I had completed cannulating and readied my drugs, the patient had a pulse and was breathing, albeit with support. We now had a solid chance of saving this guy's life. It was time to get going; the quicker the better. We deputised a few of the blokes in the bar and they helped us transfer the patient on to a trolley bed and out to the ambulance.

I took the man's brother in the car with me and we sped off to the nearest hospital. He was taken straight into Resus where the good work continued. When I left to green up, he was breathing for himself and he had fairly stable vital signs.

Our performance as ambulance personnel has led to the incredible success of CPR for more and more patients, young and old. Survival outcomes statistics continue to rise and I go to more recoveries than losses now. There still remains the high probability of failure, but that should have more to do with the predisposing clinical condition of the patient, rather than the sterling efforts of ambulance staff.

CLOSE CALLS

The worst close calls you get involve sick children. The heaviest of all weights, I think, is the one you bear when you hold the life of someone else's child in your hands. My colleagues will testify to this, especially those who have experienced the stress of working alone with a dying child until help arrived.

I sped through rush hour traffic on the way to a *'6-year-old fitting'*. Then the information was updated to state that he was no longer having a seizure and was simply *'hot'*. As I hurried to get there, my instinct was that this would be a fairly run-of-the-mill infection and temperature-related fit; in other words, non-epileptic and likely to end with me assessing a conscious and lively (albeit warm) child.

Despite this, I tried not to be complacent: it was my first call of the night shift, and there's a tendency - for some unknown reason - for the first and last calls to be bad. I got out at the given address and headed towards a door which was open and being guarded by a little girl. She had been sent to ensure I went to the correct house. She looked up at me with big brown eyes and said nothing as I walked past her and into the flat.

Inside, a woman was kneeling on the floor, phone to her ear, looking down at a little boy who was on his side, writhing and shaking. He was clearly having difficulty breathing properly and his airway was very noisy. The woman handed me the phone as I put my bags down and assessed the situation. The call-taker from EOC was on the other end and, as I unpacked what I needed, she confirmed my presence on scene and I asked her when I could expect an ambulance. I made it clear that I needed it quickly. She told me that one was on its way but I didn't get an ETA, and nor did I remember to ask her *not* to have the call downgraded or over-ridden by a higher priority whilst the crew were en-route. I knew they would have been thinking the same as I had after the information update, and I hoped that the tone of my voice had carried enough weight for an experienced call-taker to recognise that I was actually dealing with something serious.

The boy's sats - his oxygen saturation level - was extremely poor, his pulse was racing and he was hot to touch. He was in spasm, especially around the diaphragm, and was completely non-responsive. I gave him rectal diazepam to try and stop the seizure and then I got on with re-establishing his obs.

SATS. Saturation levels - specifically, oxygen saturation levels. We use a device called an oximeter to determine the amount of oxygen that has bonded to the haemoglobin. A normal, healthy person would be expected to have between 95% and 100% saturation - in other words, their haemoglobin is attracting a full complement of oxygen molecules. If the level falls below 95%, something may be amiss. Levels below 90% are becoming critical. Asthmatics may have low sats during an attack - say 93% - and will need supplemental oxygen to boost their haemoglobin levels. People with chronic breathing problems usually have permanently low sats.

His status didn't change, and his breathing was now causing me great concern. He was becoming flaccid, except for his phrenic spasms, and he wasn't getting anywhere near normal. I knew I had to get him to hospital without delay. His mother told me that he had been like this for 20 minutes and that she had been considering taking a taxi to hospital before I'd arrived.

> **PHRENIC SPASMS. These are spasms in the diaphragm, with many causes. They can be very minor - a hiccup is a phrenic spasm - or life-threatening. In this case, it was caused by seizure.**

After what seemed a lifetime, the crew arrived and I wasted no time in getting the little boy into the back of the ambulance. I cannulated him and considered another dose of diazepam, but something wasn't right with this. We set off on blue lights and I asked the attendant to put a nasal tube in. The child's breathing had now become much noisier and he was clenching his teeth - this could mean there was a problem with his brain.

His breathing began to deteriorate, despite his airway being improved by the nasal tube. He wasn't breathing adequately enough and so we 'bagged' him and prepared to resuscitate. All the time, I was reaching over to the mother, who was travelling with her daughter, to comfort her and reassure her as best I could.

When we arrived at hospital, the boy's condition had deteriorated significantly. The attendant carried him whilst the other EMT continually ventilated him. A colleague from my base station helped with the oxygen and that freed me up to begin the hand-over in Resus. I stood and related the history and my findings, including drugs given and other treatment carried out, whilst the Resus team and a paediatric registrar worked on the little boy. His mother and sister stood in isolation at the end of the room, distressed and overwhelmed.

Before I left, the team had intubated the boy and had him on a ventilator whilst they worked out what could be wrong with him. I spoke to his mother, gave her a little hug and reassured her daughter, who burst out crying from a state of staring silence. I sat with the crew who had been with me throughout this and had a cup of tea. I was shaken up inside.

Then I got a lift back to my car, which had been left on scene. I said thanks and goodbye to the crew and off I went, back to base to reset my head and complete my VDI, not knowing whether we had saved the little boy or not.

A few days later, thanks to a colleague, I received a telephone call telling me that he had survived and was back at home awaiting the results of a brain scan. A massive relief. His life had been hanging in the balance, for sure.

VDI. Vehicle Daily Inspection. Drivers of all vehicles in the Service are required to check the safety and roadworthiness of any vehicle they use. The check includes all equipment on board.

Working with sick children when you are part of an ambulance crew isn't any less stressful, but the reassurance of backup and the availability of more expert hands is valuable. We were called to a house in a quiet street for a 'two-year-old child with difficulty breathing'. Often we can expect to find nothing more than a kid with the sniffles; a lot of parents who call us with this description have misunderstood the nature of the questions asked by the call-taker, or are simply panicking because they are inexperienced or ignorant.

This time was not like that. We walked in to find the mum holding a very exhausted-looking child. He had been suffering an asthma attack for the past hour or so and, despite the fact that there was an inhaler and 'spacer' device for administering relief, both were sitting on the window ledge, unused. It turned out that the parents, who were both non-English speaking, didn't know what it was for - their GP had diagnosed asthma and given them the inhaler, but they had been none the wiser about either the diagnosis or the treatment.

There were now three of us at the house, including an FRU paramedic who had arrived first. It was clear the kid was in trouble - his breathing had become so weak that he was giving up altogether, and he needed to get to hospital quickly if he was not to die. We took him from his mother and ran to the ambulance, mum and dad running alongside. As we got going, he was treated with a nebuliser, though we knew this would do little good at this stage because he could hardly breathe the drug he needed into his lungs. As we weaved through the London traffic, sirens blaring, he looked very close to suspending, and the necessary equipment to keep him alive was made ready just in case. It wasn't needed: we got him into Resus without further deterioration and the team there began the work of stabilising him. But it looked grim. I left them fighting for his life, walking past the parents on the way out. They looked in a state of shock, completely bewildered; if only they'd understood what the inhaler was for. As is so often the case, I never found out what the outcome was.

A similar emergency for an asthmatic child in the middle of the night reinforced how important it is for us not to be complacent about *'child with DIB'* calls.

DIB. Difficulty in breathing. The term should only be used for those who are genuinely having trouble breathing in or out, or are having to struggle to breathe. Unfortunately, because the system we use prompts the call-taker to ask if someone has difficulty breathing the answer, especially for the frequent fliers and the inebriated, will invariably be YES... and that starts a whole emergency cycle, costing you (the taxpayer) millions of pounds each year. The flip side is that not to ask the question may mean that somebody with genuine DIB will slip through the net and possibly die - although the chances of that happening are much less than someone answering YES to get an ambulance quicker (and someone else who really needs it dying instead).

My crewmate and I arrived to find the FRU on scene and a little crowd of neighbours standing outside the address. There was an anxious look on each of their faces as they glanced at us.

We went into the house and the FRU paramedic was already on her way out with a very floppy child. She was running towards us, in fact. We took the hint and turned ourselves around so that we could get the ambulance ready. He was a little boy and he was hardly breathing. He was being nebulised, but it was having little effect as far as we could see. He was only four or five years old and had suffered asthma since birth. He had a history of acute severe attacks and had been hospitalised on many occasions, but his mother, worryingly, told us that this was the worst she had seen.

We took him into the ambulance and the care continued. Our drugs weren't having much effect - mild, at best - but at least they were keeping him stable. I looked at him lying in the artificial light of the vehicle; he looked as if he wanted to sleep forever, which is precisely what he was going to do if we didn't get him to hospital quickly. The neighbours moved out of the way and someone stood in the road to halt any traffic as we turned our vehicles around for the 'blue light' run to the nearest Accident and Emergency department. He was going to make it by the skin of his teeth. I had the necessary resuscitation equipment ready and strategically hidden from mum, but it would all have to come out if this child decided not to hang on any longer. Luckily, we got him to hospital in good time. He was still fighting for breath but his condition hadn't deteriorated as rapidly as it had been before treatment began and his vital signs had even improved a little. An upward curve in anyone's condition is always good news.

He survived his ordeal and was eventually discharged, but we all know that one of us will see him again and that, one day, his luck may run out.

Some close calls occur because the patient has been living with an acute problem for days, or even weeks, and has only just decided to call an ambulance. These individuals tend to be strong-willed, stubborn or just plain old-fashioned and believe in the principle of only calling an ambulance if you are at death's door. (I only wish some of our regular callers were more like that.) Unfortunately, many of them have got death's door half open by the time they, or their relatives or friends, decide enough is enough and call us out.

We went to the house of a 63-year-old man who had been complaining of problems urinating. This was a low priority call because no details of anything untoward had been given. As far as we were concerned he probably had a urinary tract infection and that was why he couldn't pee properly. Inside the house, his family gathered to explain that the man was in the toilet at that moment.

'He's having a pee now,' said his wife. 'He loses a lot of blood every time he goes.'

That didn't sound good. 'What do you mean, "loses a lot of blood?"' I asked.

'Well, he goes to the toilet every ten minutes and it's just blood that he passes.'

This concerned us greatly; we waited until another family member had got him out of the toilet and brought him to us in the front room. He was walking slowly, as if he had wet himself, and we could see a red stain on his pyjama trousers.

'I've left it there for you,' he said.

'OK,' I said. 'I'll go and have a look, but let my colleague check you out first.'

We sat him down and my crewmate checked his obs while I went to the toilet and looked at what he had passed into the bowl. It was frank blood. I mean, the toilet bowl looked like it had been badly injured and was bleeding into itself.

I went back into the living room, where my colleague was chatting to the man. He'd had some pain but not a lot and he had been like this for days, apparently. The family had thought nothing of it, at first, because he'd often had urinary problems and, in the first day or two, he'd passed only a small amount of blood each time he went to the toilet. But now his visits were much more urgent, more frequent and, as I'd seen, very bloody. He had no significant medical history to explain this development, and he was normally healthy. Now, however, he looked ill; very pale and drawn. He was also very weak on his legs. We got him into the ambulance and prepared to set off, but he insisted on sitting in the chair rather than lying on the bed, which would have been preferable.

'I'll need to go again soon,' he said, 'so I can't lie down. When I need to pee I can't help myself so it'll be difficult for me unless I'm upright.'

We relented and drove off with him sitting upright. So far, his obs were stable, but we were concerned about his blood pressure, considering the amount of blood he must have passed over recent days. We'd already decided that if it fell significantly he was going to have to lie on the bed, regardless of his urgency to go. During the journey, which was supposed to be an emergency run, he had to pass fluid, so we had to stop and he stood up in the ambulance and peed blood into a vomit bowl. He passed about a cupful and it took him a couple of minutes to complete the exercise because he found it hard to put enough pressure on his bladder to allow a full flow. The task exhausted him. We set off once more, but only a couple of minutes had passed before he needed to go again. Another stop and another cup of blood later, we carried on.

Our lights were on and the siren was being used but we were travelling at 10 mph because he repeated his stand up and pee blood routine again and again. The vomit bowl was quickly starting to fill, but we made it to the hospital just as it looked like we were going to have a bloody floor. It took us three times as long to get there as it should have - it was one of the most bizarre journeys I have taken with an emergency patient. We handed him over and left him; he was a nice old chap and I hope they got him sorted.

Doctors often call ambulances for patients who have come into the surgery with acute problems, like chest pain. They'll dial 999 without hesitation if the person they are treating suddenly becomes worse, arrives with obviously serious illnesses or injuries, needs immediate hospital care or simply presents too complex an issue for the GP to solve at that location.

A call to an 'unwell baby' at a doctor's surgery in east London had my crewmate and me, once again, preparing for the worst. The child was so obviously 'going off' that I was surprised the doctor was so laid back about it when we went to get him. His mother had no idea just how sick the child was.

'His breathing is shallow and he's not responding much,' the doctor told us.

'How long has he been like this?' I asked.

'It started about twenty minutes ago,' she replied. 'Then he was fine, then a few minutes ago he went back to being like this.'

I was feeling a little under pressure here. The child was not doing well and could suspend on us at any time. We grabbed our stuff and took him and his mother to the ambulance. I opened up the red paediatric bag that contains the specialised emergency equipment I would need if the baby stopped breathing on the way and sat down with him in my arms while the mother looked on anxiously. I supported his breathing and continually tried to stimulate a response from him, but I got very little. Mum kept asking me what was wrong with him. I didn't have a clue; neither had the doctor. All I knew was that he was in trouble.

I discovered a week or so later that the child had a serious neurological condition and was undergoing tests to see what could be done for him.

Close calls can develop as a direct result of the action, or lack thereof, taken by parents when their child presents with a possible life-threatening condition. In the middle of the night we were sent to a *'3 year-old male, fitting'*. We arrived on scene within a few minutes and made our way up to a second floor flat in a dismal estate. It was raining and cold - the weather had been like that all night and this was our last job of the shift.

Inside the dimly-lit bedsit, we found a mother crouching over her little boy whilst he appeared to be having a major seizure. There was another child in the room, lying on her back in a cot, staring at the ceiling while her brother's drama unfolded right across from her. She showed no sign of emotion or interest.

My crewmate and I approached the woman - she was African - and asked her what had happened. She didn't reply. I looked at the boy and saw that he needed help with his airway, so I cleared his mouth and nose of mucus and made to give him oxygen. His mother insisted that it wasn't necessary and tried to prevent me from putting the mask on his face. I couldn't believe what she was doing and practically wrestled with her to get the desperately-needed oxygen to her son. Eventually, she relented.

His seizure stopped but his breathing remained very noisy. I told the mother that we needed to get him to hospital quickly and I picked him up to carry him out to the ambulance - that's when I noticed something very unusual. The little boy was covered from head to foot in some kind of oil. He was slippery to hold and I nearly dropped him on the floor as I lifted him.

'What's this on his body?' I asked.

'Oil,' she said. 'It helps him get better.'

I stood and looked at her for a second.

'Oil?' I repeated.

She nodded.

'What kind of oil?'

'Olive oil.'

I was dumbfounded, and so was my partner. I know nothing of African beliefs or traditional medicines, but I do know smearing olive oil on seriously-ill kids is a waste of time. This woman had left her son suffering for so long, only calling an ambulance because she had run out of options, that she had placed him close to death. He had been fitting for a while without any medical attention whatsoever, and he was by now very unwell.

'OK,' I said. 'We need to go now. Can you arrange for someone to care for your little girl, then get your stuff ready and follow us to the ambulance?'

She nodded and left. We had to dry the poor little lad's body with paper towels before moving him because he was just too slippery to handle safely, but eventually we got him down to the vehicle where we began the process of trying to stabilise him for the journey to hospital. It only took us a couple of minutes to get ready to go, and as my colleague climbed into the driver's seat I looked around for the mother. She was nowhere to be seen.

'Hang on a sec,' I said, and hopped out of the vehicle and looked around for mum. Surely she understood the gravity of the situation? So where the hell was she? Time was absolutely critical here. I called out for her in vain. Then I heard a voice in the shadows - it was the mother chatting on her mobile phone to someone. There was no hint of stress in her voice. I called to her, and beckoned. 'Come on,' I said. 'We really need to leave now.'

She ignored me.

'Get in the ambulance now!' I shouted.

She gave me a look, hung up and walked over - still in no hurry.

We finally got going, but the little boy was getting no better. His breathing had to be supported all the way and he was in peri-arrest; this meant he could die at literally any moment. During the entire journey, the mother said nothing and showed no emotion. I sat there, 'bagging' her son to keep him alive and she stared out of the window. I felt something like disgust, but I couldn't express it.

The resuscitation of this child continued in hospital and I believe he survived his ordeal. I made an official complaint about the mother and the issue of the oil. I have no idea what happened about it. Probably nothing.

Not every close call is a life-or-death situation. There are lucky escapes which often defy the laws of physics and astound us all when we get on scene. Like the case of the luckiest Aussie I've ever met. He had fallen from the third floor window of a Bloomsbury hotel - located less than two hundred metres from my station - and I expected to be dealing with a serious head injury at the very least. In fact, I had pretty much resigned myself to the possibility that he would be dead when I got there. I raced to the scene and found a solo motorcycle paramedic attending to someone on the ground, on the other side of a fence. I climbed up onto it and leaned over, looking through the little crowd which had gathered around and trying to assess the situation. I shouted to the paramedic. 'Do you need a Delta Alpha, mate?'

He didn't answer, so I called for one anyway. I could see the guy he was attending to. He was lying on his back and he was talking, so that was a good sign. Maybe this wasn't 'as given'. I hopped over the fence and went down to where all the action was; I found myself on a narrow little patio area set aside for guests to have a drink outside. I thinned out the crowd, getting rid of anyone not connected to the guy and getting a porter to open the little gate at the end of the patio so that the crew could get access when they arrived.

Then I turned to the bloke on the ground. He had no major head injury; in fact, he had no visible injury at all. He was lying there, smiling up at his little audience with a strangely serene look about him. I looked up. Three floors was a hell of a way down. Surely he hadn't fallen from up there?

I leaned over and took a closer look. He was practically unscathed and very, very drunk. He wanted to get up, but he was being held down by the paramedic. 'I've called for a Delta Alpha,' I said.

'We're OK, I think,' said the paramedic. 'You can cancel it.' A wise choice after all, I thought.

I gleaned the story of how this young man came to be where he was from an eyewitness - a firefighter from the States. He told me that the Aussie had walked into his room unannounced, said something vague about not finding someone, and had then continued walking the length of the room and through the third floor window, falling vertically 40 feet to the patio below. He made no sound and there was no effort to save himself during the flight.

He'd landed on a metal table, which had crushed instantly. Had he landed on the concrete, he would have been killed or severely injured without a doubt. There's no doubt the table saved his life. It broke his fall and absorbed almost all of the energy, in the same way that crumple zones in car wings and bonnets take the brunt of most accidents. Luckily, there was nobody actually sitting at it when he fell from heaven. Now he was lying on the ground, surrounded by worried looking staff and concerned paramedics, with nothing worse than a scratched elbow to show for his adventure.

He was full of energy and, on reflection, it looked pretty clear to me that he had taken more than just alcohol. He was buzzing. When I spoke to him, he shook my hand and our conversation turned into a Python sketch.

'Awrite, mate?' he said. 'What's the problem?'

'You fell a long way and you might have serious injuries.'

'Nah mate, I'm awright… look!' Now he was demonstrating his full range of movement by windmilling his arms around and attempting to raise his legs.

'Yes,' I said. 'That's all very well, but you fell from the third floor window.'

'Yeah,' he said. 'I've fallen before. I've had worse.'

'It's a long way to fall, so you may have injuries you can't feel yet.'

He looked at his elbow. 'Nah… it's just a scratch, mate.'

I couldn't help smiling all the time I was talking to him, but I thought it possible he might have a head injury which was being masked by the alcohol and, possibly, drugs.

The other paramedic spoke to him. 'Listen, we're going to have to cut your top off so we can examine you properly and make sure you aren't hurt.'

At this, he turned quite angry. He wasn't having any of it.

'Listen, you ain't cutting this top off,' he said. 'It's brand new.'

'We have to cut it off so that we can examine you properly.'

'You cut this top, mate, and I'll sort you out.'

'Well, it'll be cut at hospital anyway, so why don't you let us do it?'

'No way!'

And that was that.

By now, we had more than enough resources on scene to deal with him - two ambulance crews, the solo motorcycle paramedic and me. He stretched his arms out deliberately to stop us getting him into the back of one of the vehicles, locking his elbows to make it difficult to get him past the back doors. You've done this before, matey, I thought to myself. He laughed all the time, joking at our expense.

When he got into Resus the first thing they did was cut off his top. He lay there looking very upset and suddenly very passive.

'Aww, mate,' he moaned.

I think reality was sinking in at last.

TERRORISM

On July 7, 2005, terrorists hit London again. In a big way. Not since the end of the IRA mainland bombing campaign had the Capital seen the horror of a large-scale, indiscriminate attack on innocent people, and the Provisionals had never managed anything this big.

It turned out to be a huge test - the first in some years - of the ambulance service's ability to cope.

On that day, I was at St Thomas' Hospital practising my intubation skills on people undergoing routine operations in theatre. At around 09:50 I got a call from a friend at LAS. 'There's been some sort of incident at Liverpool Street station,' she said. 'They think a train has crashed. It sounds pretty bad.'

I didn't think much of it; it wasn't as though everyone was being called in to work. But twenty minutes later, I got another call.

This time I was told that London Underground thought that there may have been some kind of 'electrical explosion', although the word 'bomb' had also been used and was now catching everyone's attention in the Control room.

There was still a lot of confusion about exactly what had taken place and on what scale, so I went back to theatre and continued my work. Just as we were preparing the next patient for her operation, the hospital's Clinical Director interrupted us. 'I'm sorry,' he said, 'but all surgery is being cancelled today.'

Obviously, this was a bit bigger than I'd first thought. The hospital around me was going into Major Incident mode, with staff hurrying here and there and little knots of people engaged in quiet, urgent discussions. I put on my uniform and got out of there as quickly as I could.

By the time I got to the ambulance station, the picture was clearing slightly. It was now evident that a number of bombs had been set off, and I was asked to join a team of medics who were heading out to one of the scenes, at King's Cross. I sat in the vehicle and the tension was palpable. No-one spoke much, and I'm sure everyone felt the same as me: nervous, concerned about what we would find, and mentally running through some of the procedures we might use.

Just before we left, I got hauled out and sent back to St Thomas' to help with liaison between the hospital and the ambulance service. I was really gutted: I wanted to be out there with my colleagues, as a soldier wants to be at the front line. Being pulled back was difficult, but I understood the need for someone to pull it all together at casualty. During the trip back there, I listened in to the radio chatter - naturally, it was all very confused but one quick sentence leapt out of the speakers and hit me in the face: 'There are a lot of people with blood on them coming out of Russell Square tube station... *make ambulances, 100.*'

I almost didn't believe what I'd just heard. *One hundred ambulances?* It made no sense. A call for 100 hundred ambulances meant that at least 100 injured people were coming out of one small tube station (later I realised that they were survivors of the King's Cross bomb). Yet the streets around us, just south of the river at the bottom of Westminster Bridge, with Big Ben just across the water, were as they are every day - calm and normal, full of people strolling along in twos and threes, chatting on their mobiles, hailing cabs. Yet we knew that a mile or two north all hell was breaking loose: the distant wail of all those sirens drifted through the air.

When I reached my assigned point, everyone was numb and quiet. By now, we knew this: three bombs had exploded on three separate tube trains, killing a large number of people and injuring many more. The first had gone off on an eastbound

Circle Line train between Liverpool Street and Aldgate, the second on a westbound Circle Line train at Edgware Road and the third on a southbound Piccadilly Line train about 500 yards from King's Cross.

I listened in to the radio, trying to blank out the noise around me, the endless wail of sirens, people shouting, phones ringing; now messages were coming across that a bus had also been blown up in Tavistock Square, and that there were a lot of casualties now coming our way. All the other hospitals - St Mary's in Paddington, University College Hospital in Euston and The Royal London in Whitechapel - were full, and it was St Thomas' turn to start taking the injured.

Almost as soon as that message ended, people started arriving on blue lights.

It was horrifying.

When I opened the doors to the first of the ambulances to arrive back, blood and water from saline drips poured out onto my boots. The vehicle floor was awash. Inside was a woman who had lost both of her legs and she was being resuscitated in the back. The paramedic was pumping on her chest, and as he did so he was pumping the blood out of her body; he couldn't stem the bleeding and perform CPR at the same time. His driver, a young trainee, was as pale as death. I looked at the injured woman and thought, *She can't survive this*. I was completely shocked later when I found out that she had.

The first few patients were in a similar condition, missing body parts and in cardiac arrest. All of the crews were ashen-faced and exhausted; they were being asked to go back again and again to carry more casualties to us. It felt like a war zone.

As things got busier, there were screams, wailing, blood and tears all around me. People were walking themselves down all the way from Central London into the A&E department with cuts and bruising and smoke inhalation. The more seriously injured had amputations, open fractures and facial burns. The hospital was struggling to cope. This became the longest day I have ever worked. It must have been all the more so for those brave ambulance crews out there, some of whom had risked their lives alongside the police and firefighters to get down to the injured and dying underground.

One of my colleagues, a paramedic biker, was first on the scene at one of the incidents. He crawled into the Tube train through a window that had been blown open and began to triage the patients. They were still sitting in their seats, dead, dying or seriously injured, all the way down that carriage; all he could do was look and count and assess who could be saved and who couldn't. The police were in the background, yelling and shouting about a secondary device, and eventually he had to climb back out. He got onto the platform and then remembered he'd left his stethoscope behind; it had been a present from his wife, so he crawled back into that quiet, dark carriage of death to fetch it.

As the day wore on, and the fear of further attacks subsided, I heard that taxi drivers were offering free rides home to emergency staff but that hotels were doubling their room prices for those who needed to stay - a disgusting act of financial piracy, I think.

I finally booked off at around 8pm, struggling home through the heavy traffic of that evening feeling drained and very sad. I couldn't get the faces of those poor injured commuters out of my head, and I couldn't contact my family to let them know I was alright because the overloaded phone networks were down. This inability to communicate had left a lot of people frantic about their loved ones. (Earlier in the day, the networks had been briefly shut down deliberately, in the City at least; mobiles can be used to trigger explosive devices, and the police feared more may have been hidden.)

Eventually, I got back, switched on the news and sat and watched the aftermath. My partner works in the ambulance service, too, and she sat with me as the enormity of this terrible day hit home. I shed a few tears, thinking of all of those people who had bought a ticket to go on a journey but had ended up dead, dying or surrounded by the dead or dying.

Next day I went back to theatre and helped prepare some of the victims of the bombings for their operations. These were broken people, and it was heart-wrenching to watch them go under: many of them panicked and didn't want to be put to sleep. One man had his mother holding his hand as he drifted off because he was so scared. He would have been in his forties. A woman with facial burns and a chest injury cried for a long time on the trolley bed as she waited for her anaesthesia. I tried to console her as much as possible; I would be the one intubating her.

Like all of the Tube bomb victims, she had filth and debris from the blasts ingrained in her skin, especially around the face. This was soot from the tunnels and dust from the carriages, blasted into the skin by the force. The injured were wearing the masks of their experiences and I could see that they had a long way to go, long after the dirt was gone, before they would begin to get over this.

As I cannulated her and the anaesthetist set to work, she turned to me, fear in her eyes.

She wanted someone to talk to before she went under. I said, 'I was there when you came out of the ambulance. You're going to be fine.' It wasn't much, but it was all I had. Then we put her to sleep and she went in for her operation.

* * * * *

Two weeks later, a second group attempted to set off their own devices on London's trains and buses. Thankfully, they were unsuccessful. It seemed incredible: our last experience with this kind of terror had left so many dead and injured, but now we had rank amateurs at work. We remained on high alert for the entire day.

The morning after the failed attempt, I was due back in theatre - we were still working our way through the 7/7 victims. I'd heard on the news that these would-be bombers had escaped: everyone was to be vigilant because the police didn't know where these people were. Bearing that in mind, as I walked toward the hospital I saw a young man sitting on the pavement with his feet in the bus lane. Buses were swerving to avoid him but he wasn't moving. He had a hood over his head, which was bowed. I was in uniform and a number of people asked if I could check him out, so I went up to him and asked him if he was alright. He looked up and nodded but didn't reply. He was a man of Middle Eastern appearance and I noticed that he had a bag by his side. He bowed his head again and ignored me.

I hate the thought of over-reacting but there were potential bombers on the loose and this guy couldn't have acted in a more suspicious way if he'd tried. I thought he looked depressed, which is how I imagined these men would feel about their failed attempts at suicide the previous day.

There was a police guard on the Tube station entrance just down the road, so I went to one of the officers and told them about this strange man. They radioed their bosses and within a few minutes the road was sealed off at either end. The traffic disappeared and the man on the pavement didn't even notice. Other police vehicles arrived and two armed officers walked towards him. As they got close they issued a challenge and the man looked up for the first time. I wasn't close enough to see his reaction.

He was asked to put his hands where they could see them and then they checked his bag, very carefully. I listened in on one of the police radios as they described what was going on up the road and then I heard someone say 'clear'.

The officer I had reported the man to approached me and told me that he wasn't a suspect.

'Why was he sitting there like that?' I asked.

'He was just waiting for the chemist's to open,' he said.

SENSORY INSULTS

I have a good constitution. I think I do, anyway. In my job, you learn to stomach almost anything, because you see and smell a lot of unpleasant things.

Of course, there's always that one thing which triggers uncontrollable gagging and the potential to vomit in everyone, no matter how well-bound they think they are. I'm proud to say that I have never thrown up on a job in front of my patient, but you do come close.

When I started working with other people's body fluids and general mess - they tend to expel aromas that range from bearable to outright offensive - I found it difficult to keep my composure; my face is a dead give-away when I am disgusted, shocked or emotionally injured. But you become acclimatized over time and with experience. For example, I got used to the smell of vomit when I was made to carry out buckets of the stuff and pour them down a toilet during a live concert at Crystal Palace years ago. After gagging and retching I simply stopped bothering and the smell (and sight) of vomit no longer troubles me too much.

A head injury at an underground station during the Christmas period tested my immunity, mind you. The man had fallen down a long flight of concrete steps and was lying, unconscious at the bottom of them. He was seriously hurt, with a significant amount of blood pooling around him, but he was breathing and he had a pulse.

My colleague and I stabilized him as much as possible and got him into the chair to be taken up to our ambulance. During this time of year we are so busy that support from a second crew or HEMS is unlikely. We tried but failed to get help, so we did what we needed to do - we roped in the Underground staff to help us carry this man all the way up the stairs to the top.

He was big and heavy. He was still unconscious, so he was unwieldy, too. His body kept trying to slump off the chair as we hauled him, one step at a time, towards the evening air. The line I had put into his vein came out when one of the staff pulled on it by accident. That caused a bit of a mess so I had to stop and re-do it. When we got him to the top and put him into the ambulance, he began to vomit violently.

I have never seen so much of the stuff come out of a single human being, before or since. The floor of the ambulance was being consumed by thick, pungent sick. He must have eaten and drunk an awful lot before his fall. It quickly became a nightmare trying to secure and manage his airway. It took both of us to pull him over onto his side while he emptied his stomach onto the floor. The smell was unbearable, but I had to stay with it for the journey. My colleague drove to the hospital and I was left in the back to manage my patient, who was still throwing up every now and then, though in ever decreasing amounts. My uniform was speckled with it, but it was my boots which bore the brunt: I couldn't decide whether to clean them or chuck them.

We spent twenty minutes shovelling the stuff out of the ambulance after that. It took another hour to get it clean enough to continue the shift. Every piece of equipment we had used, and everything within the radius of his impressive projective range, was contaminated and had to be stripped and disinfected.

It turned out that our patient had suffered a massive brain haemorrhage before he fell. He was taken to a specialist neuro centre, and the last I heard he was still alive.

Some aromas come from specific sources, such as ostomy pouching systems (colostomy bags to you and me). There are a lot of people with these fitted; those with bowel cancer, for example. They are usually well maintained, but sometimes they are ignored and we have to deal with the consequences.

I was called to an elderly ex-drug addict, now an alcoholic on two bottles of wine per day, with cancer of the bowel. He had been bleeding from his rectum (PR) and I walked into his little front room expecting to deal with a mess to begin with.

He was in bed when I arrived and his sheets and covers were filthy with his own waste. They were toxic and I have no idea how many different gases were circulating around his home but I was breathing them in.

His problem wasn't only that he was bleeding, which in itself is an ominous sign - he also had a problem with his colostomy bag. It was full, and I mean full. It was almost overflowing and smelled so foul I couldn't stay near him for more than a couple of seconds at a time. It took me a long time to get his obs.

On top of that smell, hidden somewhere in the sensory background, was the worn-in stink of cigarettes and stale food.

He was living in this every day. He rarely went out and he rarely got a visit from anyone; thus his place was a shambles.

He was not in good health, so I fought the urge to run outside until I had checked and reassured him because, despite what I have described, he was a good person and he was genuinely concerned about his life. I didn't go outside for fresh air until the crew arrived to take him away. I went out as they came up the stairs and I warned them about the olfactory hell that they were about to enter. One of the crew members was a trainee; I felt for her.

On an early morning call I was asked to investigate someone shouting for help at a railway station. I searched the area and found nobody who needed my help. Then I spotted a couple of police officers and realised they were looking for someone too. At the same time I noticed a ragged figure in a phone box and when he saw me he waved and gestured for me to stop. So I stopped and approached.

Inside the call box was a homeless old man and he had a particular problem which I could identify instantly by the smell alone. He, too, had a colostomy bag, and it, too, had over-filled and was now leaking. Watery faecal matter was running down his trouser legs and onto the ground. I had to keep him inside the phone box. He wanted to escape but I couldn't allow it - people were passing by on their way to work. The smell was outrageous, and letting it escape from the box would have been some kind of environmental violation, I'm sure.

The police officers walked over but would not go near the man. I called for an ambulance (he was not getting in my car) and I prepared myself for the apology I was going to have to give the crew when they arrived. The smell was everywhere now and the old man was complaining that he couldn't stand up any longer. I put a blanket over him and told him to sit on the ground inside the phone box. I felt cruel, but I had no choice. I couldn't allow him to wander about spreading his faeces on the street. It was rush hour and I was serious about containing this mess. People were walking past with breakfast buns in their hands, recently bought from the nearby McDonald's.

The old man began to retch and vomit because of his own stench. He had the stuff all over his fingers now. He was a health risk. I had nothing appropriate to clean him with, though even if I had he was in too cramped an environment for me to even attempt it.

The crew arrived ten minutes later and took him off to hospital. This kind of job is what really fuels my enormous admiration for nursing staff. Think about it next time you hear someone moaning about nurses, or the next time the question of their pay comes up: they have to finish cleaning up the jobs that the ambulance crews begin. That sort of smell doesn't leave your nostrils for hours, and even though the old man hadn't got in my car, for the rest of the day it smelled as if he had.

Dealing with faeces is never good. You find yourself looking out for it whenever you enter an environment where it is likely to be loose. Sometimes you find it on your gloves, or worse, your arms, as a consequence of moving or lifting a person. The elderly, incapacitated, the drunk and the mentally ill are all culprits for surprising you with their bodily waste. Obviously, it's not as if they mean to contaminate you with it, they just don't know they're in a mess.

The worst kind of faecal matter I have ever encountered is the bloody kind - 'malaena'. The word describes black, tarry faeces produced when blood is partially digested and excreted. The presence of malaena suggests bleeding into the digestive tract from, for example, cancer or a ruptured ulcer. It is taken seriously and it has one other attribute: it smells very bad.

An elderly woman had got trapped in her bath and I was asked to go and help her get out of it. By her own account, which was vague at best, she had been there for as long as three days. She hadn't actually taken a bath, because there was no water or evidence of water having been used. The mystery was how she had got herself in, why she was there and what had happened to her in there during those alleged 72 hours.

When I arrived on scene I could smell the problem from the bottom of the stairs leading to her flat. She had been found by her sisters and one of them told me that she had 'made a mess'. Sure enough, when I saw her lying in that little bath in that tiny bathroom, the cause of the offensive smell became instantly obvious. She was lying in her own waste and there was a lot of it. No part of her body had escaped contact with it. I felt so sorry for her - she was completely unaware of her situation.

Her sisters were unable to help her because they, too, were elderly. I couldn't get her out of the bath myself because she was too frail, too messy and there was nowhere to put her. I had to wait for the ambulance to arrive. In the meantime, I checked her obs and thought up a plan for her extrication; a plan that would leave me and the crew as mess-free as possible. My own arms were already contaminated.

When the crew arrived, I explained the situation and suggested we use a blanket to completely envelope the woman, making it easier to lift her out. This was the least hazardous way of removing her, I thought, but it was still going to be very tricky and messy.

We wrapped her in the blanket so that she was cocooned, and literally hauled her out of the bath and onto the ambulance carry chair. She struggled because she didn't know quite what was happening, but eventually we got her to the ambulance and on to the bed.

The cause of her malaena needed urgent investigation, but her apparent confusion about how she got where she was and how long she had been there was also a problem. I honestly couldn't see her going back to live on her own in that flat.

Blood from other orifices can provoke offensive reactions without warning too.

After a lazy morning start I was called to a man *'coughing up blood'* in a police cell. When I arrived, the police Forensic Medical Examiner (FME) introduced himself and filled me in. The guy had been brought in drunk (he was a known alcoholic) and had recently started to cough up bright red blood. 'He's produced two cupfuls so far,' said the doctor, his eyes twinkling with delight.

'Thanks,' I said. I had just eaten my breakfast, so I didn't really need to know *that* much - well, I suppose I did need to, but I'd rather I didn't.

I walked into the cell and recognised the man. He is a known homeless alcoholic whose health is questionable at the best of times. He was sprawled on the bed, looking drunk and unwell at the same time. There was a cup on the floor below him and I could see that it was full to the brim of blood and thick saliva. I had a quick look at it (I didn't want to linger on it) and questioned him briefly about his health. I carried out my obs and before I completed them the ambulance crew had arrived.

Now I was a wee bit put off by the smell, the cup full of blood and congealed saliva and the general state of the man already, but when he reached over absent-mindedly and lifted the cup to his lips, with every intention of drinking the contents, I thought I should intervene before I was left with an unappetising memory for lunch time and quite possibly the rest of the day. He was about to sip it like it was a cup of the most delicious tea.

I ran forward, shouted at him to stop and put my hand between him and the horrible contents. He looked bewildered and obviously wondered what I was playing at. As far as he was concerned this was a tipple. He was insistent at first, but I think he got the message eventually.

* * * * *

Urine has a fascinatingly changeable smell. Ordinary, run-of-the-mill urine smells like... pee. Its aroma isn't too bad, and providing the person excreting it doesn't drink the wrong liquids, it should be fairly clear and dilute. Urinary Tract Infections (UTI) turn one person's pee into another's nasal nightmare. Every day at least one ambulance crew will take someone to hospital with a UTI. In some individuals it is borderline offensive, but in others it can be an insult you never forget.

I can pretty much always now recognise a UTI with some certainty just by the smell. It is acrid and clings to every hair in your nose. In greater concentration, it would probably stain clothing and strip paint from the walls. There have been occasions where I truly believe the paint on a patient's walls *has* been removed in this way.

A call to an elderly lady who wasn't feeling well and 'not herself' and I arrived at a house where the family had gathered to worry about Grandma. She was a lovely woman but she wasn't making any sense. In fact, she was completely confused and thought I was there to take her home. Maybe she saw the analogy between an ambulance and a taxi and just put two and two together. I recognised the pungent smell of urine in the room and checked her temperature; it was high. She had an infection and I was willing to bet it was in her urinary tract.

She needed to go to hospital and an ambulance was arranged to take her. Meanwhile, she was drifting in and out of lucidity and perhaps consciousness. I didn't really want to be resuscitating her in the condition she was in because her family would never forget the scene, so I did all I could and kept her awake until a crew arrived to take her away.

Then there's the oddly numbing aroma of decaying bodies - dead, wet flesh is the worst kind of smell in my book.

One of the less attractive jobs thrust upon us is 'recognition of death'. You can be as dead as a dodo but it has to be officially recorded by someone who is qualified to confirm life is extinct; the police can't do this, and it's unlikely that their on-duty doctor will show up on scene to say 'Yep, he's dead', so the ambulance service are reeled in. Most of the time, it's a routine task and the dead person had been found within a reasonable time and is in a good condition (for a corpse, obviously). Sometimes, however, this isn't the case.

I was called to a flat in a sprawling estate to check on the status of a body that had been found by the police after a neighbour alerted them to a 'strange smell coming from underneath the front door'. That's the phrase that tells us something horrible is just the other side of the plywood.

I showed up with my crewmate and the police were happily waving us up from the third or fourth floor. We climbed the steps (why are there never any lifts in these places?) and arrived at the door of the address. One of the officers simply said, 'I don't think you're needed; he's been there for a long time.' My crewmate thought this was a reasonable summation and decided he wouldn't go in. Stupid me wanted to see what the fuss was all about.

I entered the flat and went down the dark hallway towards the front room, where a lone police officer was standing guard. I walked in and the smell hit me so hard that I couldn't see for a few seconds. It was like breathing acid into my lungs. It didn't so much provoke a need to retch as a need to douse myself in water.

On the floor there lay a lump - a human lump. It was clearly a man's body, but it was no longer defined as one. Instead, it was a heap of fly-covered flesh. It was face-down, thank God. The part of the body that was in contact with the air was mottled and wrinkled, but the part in contact with the floor had melted into a goo of putrid liquid. The head was almost gone because most of the face had collapsed inwards. It looked like his body was attempting to escape through the floor. He must have been here like this for weeks: so many people die alone, go unmissed. It's tragic.

As I left, I wondered how the neighbours had put up with the smell for so long. Perhaps they knew the truth but just didn't want to face it. I dread to think what kind of stain was appearing on the ceiling of the flat below.

HIT AND RUN

Unfortunately, these incidents are all too common. The 'hit' part ranges from a slight knock against a pedestrian's leg, to mowing someone down at high speed and killing them. The 'run' part comes when the driver leaves the scene.

If you hit someone on the road and fail to stop and report it, the maximum penalty the law allows is six months in prison or a fine. (As a comparison, you can go to prison for life for robbery.)

It's scary how common it is. I read a piece recently in *The Daily Telegraph* which said that the most recent UK hit and run statistics (for 2004) showed 23,714 incidents, which resulted in personal injury to over 28,000 people, 145 of whom died.

I have tried to understand the mentality of drivers who 'run', but I guess until I am in the situation myself I don't know how I'm going to react. Well, actually, that's not true. I'm sure I'd do the right thing, regardless of the consequences to me, which explains why I struggle to understand those who don't.

Could be the car is stolen, or the driver is uninsured (there are currently over a million of them on the roads). Alcohol may have something to do with it. There may be illegal drugs in the vehicle, or perhaps the driver has a previous criminal conviction. I think some of them are just plain stupid. A minority probably think they will get away with it and hide out at home for a while.

Many times, the injuries are horrible.

I received an early morning call to a Road Traffic Collision (RTC) in the West End. It was evening rush hour, it was dark and raining and the traffic was hell. I was a mile or so away. The call details stated *'vehicle vs. ped. - ?inj'*.

Nothing could have been further from the truth than *'? inj'*.

After battling through the traffic, sirens and blue lights going, I arrived at the scene and found it cordoned off by the police. I'd been expecting someone, possibly drunk, to have been superficially injured after bumping lightly into a parked vehicle. We get that end of the RTC market, too. The cordon put paid to those thoughts. This meant that it was a serious incident. I continued down the road until I got to the scene. There was an ambulance in attendance but I couldn't see the crew or the casualty. Two buses were blocking my access to the area and the bus drivers, who were parked side by side across the entire road, were having a conversation and not paying any attention to my flashing blue lights. I sounded my siren and they looked. A police officer waved at them and one of the guys climbed aboard his bus and moved it out of my way. I drove around the wrong side of the road to the accident scene.

I parked up and glanced over my shoulder at the road behind me. One of my colleagues was attending to a casualty on the ground. Then I realised what I was seeing. A young woman, in her early twenties, lay in the middle of the wet road with a large pool of blood around her. Her red-soaked clothing had been cut open, so she was lying on it and exposed to the air and the rain. We always do this with serious injuries because we need to inspect the body; we also need access to skin for defib pads.

His crewmate rushed back from the ambulance with some equipment as I got out and ran over to them.

This young woman was in serious trouble. She had a massive and very obvious head injury: the whole left side of her face had been obliterated. She lay there and her legs and arms moved in a grotesque slow-motion mime for help. I have no idea whether she understood what was happening to her or not; all I do know is that she squeezed my hand once when I spoke to her but that she didn't respond like that again afterwards.

Someone had hit her hard and had left the scene. A coward with a car as a weapon had wiped this young girl's future out in a split second and hadn't had the guts to stay and help her. Nobody witnessed this apparently and she had been lying in the middle of that road for God knows how long, with her life bleeding onto the street, until somebody saw her and called for help.

All her personal belongings were strewn around her and we worked frantically to keep her alive. To be honest, I expected her to die on us in the road, but miraculously she was staying, just hanging on by the thinnest of threads.

Another FRU arrived and the four of us gathered her up in the scoop and got her into the ambulance. The oxygen mask didn't sit properly on her face because of the extensive damage and intubating her (if it became necessary) would be almost impossible. I had called for an emergency doctor to attend but it was going to take too long for him to get here; she had us and we weren't waiting. I gave her a large dose of morphine before we set off.

In the ambulance fluids were given and, as well as her more obvious injuries, a left side pneumothorax was identified.

> **PNEUMOTHORAX. The lungs are lined with a double membrane separating them from the chest wall. A pneumothorax involves air getting between these two membranes, which causes the lung to collapse and makes breathing difficult.**

An attempt was made to de-compress - we use a large bore needle, inserted into the chest to get the air out of the chest cavity, which allows the lung to re-inflate and is a potentially life-saving technique - but it was too difficult to deal with immediately, so we had to leave it. She was fighting for her life and continued to breathe, albeit agonally - agonal breathing is weak, near-death breathing - until she got to hospital. There she was put to sleep and intubated (RSI) so that her breathing could be managed properly - we'd simply not had the time to do this on scene or en route. When I left, she was still being worked on and I had no idea whether she would come through.

Amazingly, this woman beat the odds after a long stay in hospital. Her life will never be the same, but she survived one of the most horrific head injuries I have seen on a living person.

I don't know whether the evil scumbag who hit her and left her was ever caught, but I hope it's on his or her conscience. I felt terribly angry after that job, and that anger is still with me. Alongside it, though, there is a feeling of some satisfaction. What my colleagues and I did to keep her alive worked. She would have been dead within minutes without our aggressive intervention.

. Not all hit and run incidents result in such horrific injuries. They range from immediately fatal to very minor cuts and bruises (and sometimes nothing at all), but the mechanisms for injury are similar in every call of this nature and so we tend to treat all those patients with the same precautions for their spine. They get a collar around their neck and blocks by their ears before being unceremoniously strapped to a rigid board or orthopaedic stretcher (scoop).

A taxi hit a young man who stepped into its path on a rainy afternoon. He wasn't looking where he was going and, by his own admission, was completely to blame. I guess he was so relieved not to have been killed that he couldn't absolve the driver of guilt quick enough. The driver, meanwhile, was sitting on the kerb in a daze, worried sick about how badly he may have hurt the man.

In the end, even though we strapped him down and took the necessary precautions as usual, he didn't have a scratch on him. His leg may have been damaged but there was no sign of it when I examined him. The taxi had hit him at around 30mph - in a 30mph zone, that's the speed they *all* say they were doing.

'How fast were you travelling when you hit the pedestrian, sir?'

'Oh, I dunno. What's the posted limit for this street, officer?'

'It's 30mph.'

'Yes, now I think about it, that's the speed I was moving at.'

There's no point in trying to glean a confession for speeding because it just won't happen. Unless, of course, the whole thing was witnessed by credible people or is on camera.

Like the case of the small car and the large man. He was hit whilst crossing a busy road by one of those little 'easy to park and put in your pocket later' cars. When I arrived, he was sitting among a small crowd who had gathered to tend to him on the pavement. A Good Samaritan had dragged him out of the road before something else small and vicious had a go at him.

The driver of the car had screamed on around the corner, parked up (they are very easy to park) and legged it. The whole thing was witnessed, from beginning to end, by at least ten taxi drivers who just happen to congregate at that spot for a bit of a chat and a brew.

The patient was taken to hospital with a minor head injury and a possible fractured hand but was otherwise unhurt. The taxi-driving witnesses reckoned the car was doing at least twice the legal limit.

Some people simply bounce off the bumper of the car that has left them lying in the road. Usually, alcohol has influenced the outcome and their rubbery response to a 30mph impact by a ton of vehicle has left no impression on them whatsoever. This flies in the face of all we are taught on mechanisms of injury and sticks two fingers up at my school physics teacher, much as we used to during class.

A Polish drunk who got hit by a car which sped off afterwards had to be tracked down when he, too, left the scene. We had been called to the incident by police, but the victim was nowhere to be seen - witnesses said that he had been hit hard enough to send him flying but that he had then just got up and wandered off, shouting a few Polish phrases after the disappearing vehicle.

We found him staggering down an alley way behind an estate. He was still drinking and verbally abusive when we asked him to stop so that we could check him out. In broken English he told us that he didn't need our help and that he had no intention of going to hospital. A cursory check (that's all he would allow and only then because the police were present) of his obs and physical condition seemed to verify that he was unscathed by his journey through the air.

On his insistence, which was often less than gracious, we left him alone and no further action was taken as far as I am aware. Neither did we hear from our Polish friend again.

A 31-year-old Frenchman who was allegedly hit by a black cab, which subsequently left the scene, sat on a bus stop bench with British Transport Police (BTP) taking care of him until I arrived. It was 3 o'clock in the morning and the streets were all but deserted; somehow this guy had managed to get his head bashed in by one of the few fast-moving vehicles around. I mean, he must have *tried*, almost. The rest of his body was fine but he had a significant head wound.

I carefully removed the loose dressing that had been applied by the BTP and looked at his injury. A long, meandering laceration worked its way along his scalp, from his eyebrow to the middle of his head. The flesh had been completely torn away, exposing the skull underneath, yet he sat there joking about having a 'bad headache'. He wasn't drunk and he hadn't taken drugs. He had just finished a long shift and had been drinking Red Bull all night. Maybe it has an analgesic property they don't tell us about in the ads; if he'd had the wings, I think he would have been more than happy to have flown off and gone to bed.

The more I looked at him, the more I couldn't figure out how he'd got this one nasty injury and nothing else. Maybe only the wing mirror had hit him, but then the wing mirror of a black cab isn't high enough to have done this, unless he had bowed his head as he crossed the road and the vehicle had clipped it. Perhaps he had actually been hit by something with a much higher wing mirror - a bus, for example. I didn't think he was high enough on Red Bull to mistake a bus for a cab, so I dismissed *that* theory. He could, I suppose, have sustained that injury when he hit the ground after being thumped by the taxi, but there was no tell-tale pool of blood on the road or pavement. As I examined the wound it bled profusely and I had to re-dress it quickly to get the bleeding under control, so there would certainly have been a little puddle somewhere if he had lain on his head for any period of time... but there wasn't. The blood-puddle fairies had been.

He was wearing his iPod, and that gave us a useful clue. He was probably listening to music and not watching for traffic as he crossed the road. He could have been 'side-swiped' by a vehicle if the angle was just right, so his body wouldn't be involved, thus the isolated head injury.

He remained stable and in good spirits as he was taken off to hospital. His scalp flap would need to be closed properly, and he would probably need specialist treatment for some time afterwards to ensure it healed fully. He was a strange, happy, injured Frenchman, and he made treating someone who had 'gotten away with it' a pleasant experience for a change.

I know I will deal with many more hit and run incidents, and not all of them will be survivors. I know I'll face the task of keeping someone together until a crew arrives to help me out, and I know that it will happen some day soon, but I'll remind myself of the incredible difference we make to the patient's chances of survival once they are in our care. That way, it's easier to accept the aftermath of such incidents.

STREET PEOPLE

This job can play with your sense of humanity sometimes.

We meet so many people over the course of a career that we set distances according to who we think we like and those we automatically dislike, sometimes just because of their circumstances. I grew up on a council estate and had a very working-class childhood; now I dislike anything that reminds me of that. I think it's human nature to feel that way, and working with the homeless as a pre-hospital professional presents the same barrier. It becomes too easy to forget that these people have had lives before all of this, and that not all of them have abused those lives by drinking or using drugs to excess. Many homeless people are ex-soldiers, for instance, guys who've fought for their country but find it impossible to readjust to life in Civvie Street after their service has ended. But even rough sleepers who seem deserved of their fate require a pause for thought.

The charity CRISIS estimates, based on Government figures, that there are as many as 400,000 homeless adults in the UK. A large proportion of these are single homeless people, who are not entitled to any accommodation in England and Wales unless deemed to be 'vulnerable'. This gives them less incentive to apply for accommodation and they end up sleeping rough on the streets. In Scotland, the same individuals would be entitled to temporary accommodation, and from 2012 will get permanent accommodation. I can see a big shift in the homeless population to northern climes in the near future, unless the inclement weather is a problem for them.

The vulnerability of those with ongoing health problems is plain to see out there on the streets. There are individuals

Street People

suffering some of the worst illnesses there are but, although the
country's healthcare system applies to them as much as to
anyone else, access and treatment monitoring can be
impossible.

I was sent to a 41-year-old homeless alcoholic who had
been found semi-conscious and coughing up blood. He was
lying on the steps of a church that gives refuge to the local
alcoholics and drug addicts. The parish takes responsibility for
feeding them, clothing them to some extent and giving them a
place to lie down, and thank God they do.

I knew this man. He had been a patient of mine the previous
year and he had been drunk and abusive. Now he was too ill to
raise a snarl, too out of it to care. He was still drunk, and he
was lying in his own filth. There was an eye-stinging smell of
urine about him - I had to hold my breath several times to deal
with it - and he clearly wasn't well. His body needed to go to
hospital, even if his soul was meant for somewhere else.

His buddies were sitting around him and all of them showed
genuine concern. There was a sense of community among
them, as if they all looked out for each other. Of course, a few
of them were drunk and could barely keep themselves upright
when demonstrating the extent of their anxiety, but I sensed
they were used to being ignored and vilified; one of them, a
woman who looked 50 but was probably in her 30s, said: 'We
are good people, but we're alcoholics.'

It stopped me in my tracks. I could hear her, in my head,
saying, 'We get treated like crap all day… please don't do it to
him now.'

I had no intention of treating them any differently to anyone
else, but I could understand her concern.

The ambulance arrived and the man was taken away to
hospital, with the thanks of the other homeless people
following in the air. I packed up my gear and walked to the car,
and as I got in the woman shouted out to me.

'I didn't know what else to do,' she said. 'I'm sorry I called you, but I didn't want him to wake up dead.'

London Street Rescue, a comparatively new charity, sends its people out and about to 'rescue' those rough sleepers who wish to have some kind of roof over their heads (they don't all want this). They target the most vulnerable and have asked the ambulance service to work with them to help eliminate the problem. We are asked to identify people that we come across in our working day (or night) who may be vulnerable and therefore deserve rescuing. We call the charity, give some details, including the whereabouts of the individual concerned, and leave it to them. They send an outreach worker to find them and arrange emergency accommodation, give advice and information about available support services, provide blankets and food or put them back in contact with their families where possible. All in all, a good thing.

The statistics for the number of rough sleepers in the Capital are difficult to get and more often than not are woefully out of date. Ever since Ken Livingstone's initiative in the early 2000s, officially accurate figures for the reduction of street people, which he planned to reduce dramatically, have been strangely elusive. The only useful source I could find was The Simon Community, one of the oldest homelessness charities.

In April 2006, The Simon Community sent its own people out onto the streets to record the actual number of rough sleepers. This is not an easy thing to do, considering the introverted nature of some of these individuals and the inaccessible places in which they choose to bed down for the night. Nevertheless, they concluded that there were 332 people sleeping rough in London. They also phoned round the 66 hostels in Central London and discovered that there were 42 free bed spaces available but not being utilised.

One of the ways that street people make a living is by selling *The Big Issue*. In turn, the magazine uses its profits to raise funds for homelessness projects and is a registered charity.

There is, as you'd expect, fierce competition for your money and *Big Issue* sellers seem to have appeared on every street corner. To get an edge on sales, some of them have adapted 'skills' to attract your attention and hopefully your loose change. I know of a man who stands on one leg, holding out a copy of *The Big Issue* with an outstretched arm. He will stand like this for a very long time until someone takes the bait. Even more impressive is the man who stands on his head and can stay that way forever (seemingly) in an attempt to persuade you to part with your free cash.

I think there needs to be another way for these people to earn a crust. If they can't get rid of their papers maybe that's because the interest of the general public has waned and a new approach is needed. They don't want charity - for that they would simply beg (and get arrested) - but they do want the means to earn their day's food and lodgings.

* * * * *

Not all of the people who live on the street are pleasant. Not all of them care about what we are trying to do. Some of them deliberately abuse us.

I was called to attend a known patient who wears a surgical mask over his face for tuberculosis (TB), though he doesn't really need it because he doesn't have TB. He uses this as an excuse to get to hospital, where he can get free food and abuse the staff when they ask him to leave. When I got on scene, the ambulance crew were just getting to him ahead of me and so I stuck around to see what was what. He didn't have any problems and considered his imaginary TB to be enough of an excuse to go to hospital. The crew were wise to him and he was told to get a bus. I didn't disagree, I have to say; he would make his own way and we could free up an ambulance. He toddled off with his mask on, scaring the general public as he made his way to the crowded bus stop. Once he thought he was out of sight, I saw him take his mask off. He obviously decided to end the charade.

The first time I met this guy he was lying on the grass outside a busy train station, extorting sympathy and worried looks from the general public. He had collapsed and caused a scene, which included the use of his face mask, in order to get some kind soul to call an ambulance. Of course, there were many who obliged, partly out of fear of whatever it was that might be so dangerous as to warrant the barrier on his face.

I was sucked in by this because I didn't know him at the time, so I assumed he was a rough sleeper with a genuine medical problem (I was naïve in those days). He was filthy and unkempt. He had a long, shabby beard which trapped his saliva during spitting sessions, so it was sticky and wet, and he mumbled when he spoke, so I had no choice but to get close to him to hear. His breath wasn't great. It was quite unpleasant, but thankfully the hospital was only a few minutes away.

We took him in to A&E and I did my paperwork before leaving. As I climbed into my vehicle, a highly amusing scene unfolded in front of me. He was so smelly that the staff had decided it was best to have him sit in a wheelchair outside until someone could clean him up. He wasn't happy with that and promptly wheeled himself back inside. Then he was wheeled back out, this time applying resistance to the wheels in an effort to thwart the expulsion. I watched a nurse wagging her finger at him, clearly telling him to stay put, or else. As I left, he was sitting in the chair, beady eyes above the mask daring anyone who passed by to get close. On the upside, he may even have acted as an effective deterrent to anyone else hoping to turn up and waste the hospital staff's time.

Another regular caller had me out on a CAT A emergency because he was 'coughing up blood'. When I got on scene I could see no evidence of this. He wasn't weak and he wasn't ill. He was just cold and homeless. I took him to hospital myself and when I booked him in the staff told me he had walked past the hospital to make the 999 call for an ambulance (to take him where he had already been). Remember, we are all paying for this, and apart from the cost it uses up medical resources which might actually be needed.

I have noticed that street people have extremely well-behaved dogs. It must be the bond created when you have to rely solely on one person to feed you and keep you warm. There is one particular young man that I know from regular sightings who uses this to his advantage. His dog is trained to lie on its back with a baby's dummy in its mouth. Sometimes he will adorn its head with one of those frilly baby caps for additional emotional impact. The result is that lots of people, especially women - more especially, drunken women - will stop and pay attention to the animal as he lies there waiting to be stroked and cuddled. Then they part with a few quid to ensure that the dog and his master remain well-fed and healthy. I have never seen this man drunk and I have never had a call to him. He lives on the street and begs for money for food and basic comforts. I'm positive the dog is well-fed because street people take good care of their dogs.

Another regular street person became an acquaintance of mine over a two-year period, though I haven't seen him for a while. He used to sleep in the entrance to one of the large cinemas on Leicester Square, but he can no longer do that since they have completely refurbished it and turned it into a casino. I'm not sure the door staff would appreciate him turning up with his sleeping bag and settling down for the night as punters weave past to get to the debt machines downstairs.

He has a long white beard and looks older than he is (the street will do that to you), but he is a very intelligent and reserved man. He only started speaking to me when he felt he could trust me, and that only came about because I used to check that he was OK if I was passing the Square. I'd seen him having trouble with the local drunken yobs a few times before.

During one of our conversations, he told me that someone had broken his leg while he was sleeping. He didn't elaborate on how it was done, but I'm assuming they simply jumped or stamped on it. He has a permanent limp and is in constant pain as a result, but he still prefers to live on the streets. He's been doing it for over 20 years - it must be a difficult thing to get out of. It wouldn't work for me, but for some the concept of a roof overhead, and all the associated ties and bindings, must seem less and less appealing as time goes on.

Many people on the streets are vulnerable to attack - my younger brother still bears the scar from a knife slash to his face, carried out while he was sleeping in an arcade in Soho. (He slept rough when he first moved down south.)

Many of our calls to rough sleepers involve incidents in which an assault has taken place, either because of a dispute over a 'patch' or sleeping area or simply because there are some very bad people out there. Rough sleepers get killed, too.

I knew of two young girls, Kerry and Jane. Both were aged about eighteen, and they were nice girls who had ended up on the street and got involved in prostitution. I had treated Kerry, but Jane I knew only by sight. They were part of the regular cast of characters you get used to seeing if you work a patch over a period of time, though to most of the tourists and office workers passing by they were probably invisible. After a while, they just disappeared and I didn't see them around. Then I saw one of them, Kerry, the girl I'd treated in the past, sitting on the steps of a train station. The radio was quiet, so I went up to her. 'How are you?' I said. 'And how's your friend?'

'She's dead,' she said, with a deadpan face and a flat voice. 'They found her in the river.'

She then related a terrible story, one which I had read about in the papers but hadn't associated with either of these young women. Her body had been fished out of the Thames a few months back and she was found to have been brutally murdered, probably by someone she had gone with when she was 'working'. Her body had been dumped in the river soon after. It was a while before anyone noticed she was missing, and her corpse was only found by accident.

'Oh,' I said. 'Right.' I was shocked, and found myself unable to say anything remotely useful considering the horror of it. Still, here was the other girl, sitting on these steps waiting for her new friend so that they could go to work again. During the time of Jack the Ripper, prostitutes in the East End continued to ply their trade because, for many of them, the risk of death was outweighed by the necessity to find money for food and shelter. It's ironic that such a young person should be exposed to an event like this and still view her life with the same cold logic that her predecessors did over a century before.

FAKERS

I've discussed hoax callers and timewasters at length but there is one group of individuals who just can't help calling us out for their 'emergencies'. These people usually have nothing wrong with them - nothing physical anyway - and suffer instead from the desperate need for attention, particularly the attention of medical professionals. This impulse becomes an obsessive clinical condition known as Munchausen's Syndrome.

People with this condition act as if they have a physical or mental problem, when they have actually caused the symptoms themselves. They like to be seen as ill or injured, and will even undergo tests and operations, many of them painful or risk-laden, in order to get the sympathy and attention given to people who really are ill. Named after Baron von Munchausen, an 18th century German who liked to tell tall tales about his life and experiences, we also know it as 'hospital addiction syndrome'.

I have come across a number of cases over the years. In central London there are a few 'regular' culprits, well-known to the hospitals they frequently visit. Unfortunately, there isn't a list available for us to refer to so that we can identify these people when we first encounter them. Nobody tells us who is faking and who isn't, so we treat these patients in the same way as all the others, even to the point of administering drugs and pain relief for problems that don't exist. You don't need a medical degree or 15 years' experience as a paramedic to see how dangerous this can be.

My crewmate and I were called to a man who had 'severe chest pain' in Piccadilly Circus. He had been taken to the little police office located at the end of Shaftesbury Avenue where he was being helped by the police. When we arrived, we found him rolling around on the floor, apparently in utter agony and deathly pale. Between yelps and gasps, he told us he had a history of heart problems. The police officers were convinced he was going to have a heart attack and die where he was.

We took him into the ambulance and I went through my usual procedures with him. Once I'd established the scale of his pain (we use a number system, where '0' is no pain and '10' is the worst pain), I cannulated him and gave him some morphine. He had also been given an aspirin and some Glyceryl Trinitrate (GTN) spray but nothing seemed to be helping him.

> **GLYCERYL TRINITRATE works by making the veins and arteries relax and dilate. This reduces the resistance within the blood vessels and makes it easier for the heart to pump blood around the body.**

His ECG looked normal, if a little erratic, and his other vital signs were within normal limits. I was starting to wonder what was going on with the man. His pain was real enough (or so I believed) and he had a cardiac history (or so he said) - although that didn't make sense, given the normal ECG. I was confused. We took him to hospital, on blue lights and sirens, and we were inside the Resus room within a few minutes. The doctors and nurses were dealing with him using their own protocols for acute chest pain and it all seemed to be going smoothly. He was about to be given another dose of morphine when one of the nurses did a double take and pulled the doctor to one side and said something quietly. She then turned to the patient and it quickly became apparent that she recognised him and that he was *not* having chest pain - he was faking it. I've never learned to this day how he managed to look so pale.

During the course of my experiences with these people, I began to understand how much skill was involved in creating a truly believable illness - so credible, in fact, that experienced ambulance crews were more than likely going to treat them as real without hesitation. However, there are hints - things they say or do that will alert you to the possibility of a Munchausen patient.

I was on stand-by at Leicester Square when I was approached by a member of staff from one of the big cinemas there. 'We've got a bit of an emergency going on in here,' he said, jerking his thumb behind him. 'We just wondered if you could nip in for us?'

They'd called an ambulance and then seen me, so I called it in and made my way on foot to the cinema. Inside, I was directed to a man who was slumped in the aisle between seats up in the 'Dress Circle'. The film had been stopped and there was a small and uneven audience around me, a few dozen people shuffling nervously about, looking in my direction and waiting for a major drama to unfold. Off in the other rows, I could hear sweets and popcorn being munched and a buzz of low, unconcerned chatter.

The man in the aisle looked completely out of it and would not respond in any way to my questions. He was breathing, albeit slowly, and it was hard to find a pulse in his wrist. I checked his carotid (neck) pulse and it was strong. He looked to me as if he had suffered a stroke. His limbs were limp and one of his pupils was bigger than the other (although this can mean nothing at all). He was fairly big and had wedged himself in between the seats at an awkward angle, half-twisted with his lower body sticking out onto the steep stairs of the balcony area.

I busied myself with my usual checks, including blood glucose, which is always a good start with sudden collapse, and blood pressure, but nothing was amiss. All the time, I was aware of the eyes boring into me from all directions in this quiet cinema. All chatter had stopped now and everyone was looking over.

I was there for fifteen minutes before the crew arrived because the job had been categorised as a low priority for some reason. When they turned up, I had exhausted all of my checks and tests. He was still breathing and he still had a pulse but he wasn't responding to a thing I said or did. He remained floppy and heavy.

We moved him, clumsily at first, from the cinema to the ambulance and I continued my care with the help of the crew. As I tried to put a cannula in (which was tricky) he became more alert (the oxygen, I figured) and he began to speak a little.

He didn't give his name or details but he did name his 'usual' hospital, which was further south of the river than we were taking him. This was Clue 1.

I also noticed that his arms were badly scarred and that some of the scars were perfectly straight. This was Clue 2.

The scarring was the main reason I found it so difficult to find a decent vein, the tissue was so tough and it was clear that his veins had been 'got at' many times in the past so they were uncooperative. This was Clue 3.

'Are you a self-harmer?' I asked.

Not a word. He was back to his previous slumped and unresponsive self.

Just as we were about to set off on a routine journey to hospital, with me following in the car, the crew reported that his breathing had become noisy and his level of consciousness had dropped. I re-checked him as the crew tended to his airway but I couldn't find anything different in his vital signs; no blood pressure changes, no ECG variation, nothing. We decided to 'blue' him into hospital just in case.

When we arrived he was taken immediately to Resus. Again, all the usual tests were carried out and the doctors worked around him frantically. An anaesthetist was requested, to intubate him and stabilise his airway, and I went off to help with the paperwork.

When I got back into Resus 20 minutes later to check on him, I heard the nurse shouting his name (apparently) and trying to get him to respond. I listened more closely.

'Come on, Steven,' she was shouting. 'Wake up. It's time to go home now!'

Unorthodox, I thought.

Then I twigged. She knew who he was, and she was thoroughly unconcerned. She'd cancelled the anaesthetist and continued her attempts to wake him up, but he was having none of it.

'Who is he?' I asked.

'He's well known,' she said. 'He's just pretending. If you have a look at his records you'll see he does it a lot.'

You're torn between feeling sorry for these people - they clearly have *something wrong* with them, it's just not anything that an ambulance and A&E can sort out - and getting angry. What if a kid had been knocked down a few feet from where I'd been on stand-by? It might have taken several minutes for another crew to get there.

Some Munchausen patients make it easy for you to make your mind up: they can be unpleasant and demanding, using the ambulance service and the hospital staff like crutches for their emotional needs and becoming petulant and rude when they don't get what they want.

I was working an early shift on an ambulance with a colleague when we received a call to a 'known' patient complaining of chest pain. When we got there, we found her in her front room remonstrating with the FRU paramedic who had arrived earlier.

'I want to go to the Royal Free!' we heard her shout as we walked in.

'The crew will take you to the nearest A&E, that's how it works,' replied the FRU medic.

My crewmate and I accepted the hand-over for this patient and immediately got embroiled in the argument she was currently running with the FRU guy.

'I have chest pain,' she said, almost stamping her feet. 'I have a heart problem and I want to go to the Free!'

The Royal Free Hospital was a long way off compared to the nearest, which was University College Hospital (UCH). Unless there is a clinical reason for us to divert to a particular care centre, we must - for very obvious reasons - take the patient to the nearest one if it is an emergency call.

'If you have chest pain, we have to go to the nearest hospital,' my colleague said. 'I'm afraid you can't just demand to be taken to one of your choice.'

I got the impression that the woman was an old hand at this, and that the arguments she was perpetuating had been rehearsed and used many time before on different crews - crews who had perhaps relented and taken her where she wanted to go. My colleague was becoming exhausted with the fight.

'Look,' he said. 'Why don't we get you into the ambulance, check you out properly and then we can decide on where to go. Is that fair?'

I thought it was very fair and the loud woman calmed down and agreed.

We took her out to the ambulance, checked her ECG, gave her pain relief and prepared to go to hospital. We never mentioned which one she would be taken to and I drove to the only hospital that was an option - UCH.

All the while, she flopped and rolled around in the back, determined to make us realise she was in pain, despite the analgesic gas she had been taking. She could have won an Oscar, honestly; unfortunately for her, she was so caught up in the role that she didn't notice where she had been taken as we wheeled her into Resus.

She moved from the trolley to a cubicle bed, looked around, blinked a few times, and then recognised a few people (nurses she didn't like).

Furious, she started screaming at the top of her voice. 'This isn't the f**king Free,' she yelled. 'This is the f**king UC-f**king-H!'

On and on she went, suddenly and miraculously cured of all that chest pain. Finally, realising she was getting nowhere, she tore off her blanket, threw away her oxygen mask and stormed out of the hospital. She turned right, realised that was the wrong way and did an about-turn. We watched as she walked back past the glass doors with a finger raised in our direction and out into the cold morning air. She still had her nightgown on.

BELLS AND WHISTLES

Lights and sirens. We use them to alert traffic to our presence. We use them to let *you*, the pedestrian, know that we are there and to be aware of us. We use them to let worried relatives know that we are on our way and will be with their ill or injured loved one imminently. We *don't* use them to annoy you and, contrary to what many believe to be true, we never use them 'just to get home earlier'.

The blue lights are designed to be seen from a long way off. There are usually more intense strobes at the front of the light bar, so that you can tell in which direction the emergency vehicle is travelling; in other words, is it coming towards you?

On most of our vehicles, there are three main siren tones. These are activated when the '999' button is pressed on the control pad in front of the driver. In my FRU car, that pad is to my right at the level of the windscreen.

The first sound emitted is the 'wail' - that's the long, drawn-out tone. It's used on long stretches of road, to give forward warning to drivers and pedestrians ahead that we are coming. It will increase in volume as we draw closer, then it will decrease in volume and the pitch will 'bend' as we pass by. This is known as the Doppler Effect, and that's a whole different book.

There is a little 'stalk' with a button at the end, near the steering wheel, and this is used to change from one type of siren to the next. When it is pressed, the second sound is emitted and this is known as the 'yelp', which sounds like a whooping noise. This sound is more effective when approaching traffic at a junction, or in built up areas once the wail has pre-warned everyone that we are coming. It's more of an 'OK, we're here now' sort of sound. It has a faster cycle time so tends to make heads turn - especially heads that paid no attention to the first sound, or driving heads attached to mobile phones.

Finally, the 'ray gun' sound. It's not actually called that but I don't know for sure what its real name is so that's what I call it. (Some vehicles don't have this sound and instead have a 'hi-lo' option, which is similar to the old-fashioned 'nee-naw' sound but kind of sexed-up.) The ray gun sound is a harsh, rapid-cycling tone that really wakes people up. It's effective at close range when the other two sirens have failed to have an effect. It is also a transitional tone for letting traffic know that we are still on the move. The 'hi-lo' is used in much the same way but can be sounded over a long distance with much the same effect as the wail.

There is a fourth sound - the horn, which sounds like a tug boat is coming in to harbour. It's an American feature, I believe, and most of our newer ambulances, including the cars, have them fitted. At the push of a button, my Vauxhall Zafira can sound like an articulated lorry. Basically, it says, 'Get out of my way 'cos you're on my front bumper now.'

On older ambulances, the switch for changing from one siren to the other is on the floor, near the foot brake. The driver simply moves his foot onto it, clicks down and the sound will change. It also operates as the 'on-off' switch for sirens, which allowed for some hilarious pranks among ambulance staff when we all drove them. You could go into someone's parked vehicle, switch on the siren (it won't sound if the engine's off) and then run away and hide until your friend returned, ready to drive off. As soon as he or she started the engine, the siren would blare, usually in an area where the sound would be greatly amplified. The look on the driver's face was priceless and if you were good at keeping a straight face, and maybe adding a dash of concern, she or he would never know who was responsible. At any rate, they could never prove it.

Some people ignore all of our bells and whistles; it's as though it puts their backs up. But the use of light and noise isn't so much a 'move, or else' as a 'please let me pass', and it could mean we meet our target response time, or that we save someone's life. That 'someone' might just be your mum, or your husband, or your son or daughter. Any delay caused by obstructive traffic or stupid people will inevitably have an effect on our targets, or the patient's life, or both. How would you feel if you had to wait an extra minute or two with your dying loved one just because some driver didn't want to move over?

There is still an element of courtesy about moving aside for an emergency vehicle, but it is now against the law to obstruct them (or us as individuals) from performing our duties. The Emergency Workers (Obstruction) Act 2006, which came into force on February 20, 2006, makes it a specific offence to obstruct or hinder emergency workers (including ambulance personnel) who are responding to emergency calls. Currently, the maximum penalty is a fine of £5,000.

Obstructing the free movement of an ambulance in such a way as to cause a delay would be an offence under this new law, but there is confusion among drivers about what they can and cannot do when an emergency vehicle is approaching, so here are some tips to help:

*As soon as you see us and it is safe to do so, indicate and pull over to the left. We will generally drive on the outside of traffic so will want to pass you on the right. If you pull to the right, we will have no choice but to cut in to the left and this may cause an accident.

* If we approach up the middle of a lane, pull over to the left if you are driving in the left lane or the right if you are driving in the right lane. We are 'splitting you up' to make a path through the congestion.

* Do NOT stop dead in front of us. Your flashing hazard lights won't prevent an accident. You must try to avoid using your brakes unnecessarily when you see us coming. Oh, and stay off your phones while driving. I've had a number of near-misses when drivers didn't or couldn't hear my siren as I approached and then decided to pull a stunt when they suddenly saw me there. While I'm on this subject, how can you afford to be driving that three-litre monster anyway when it's clear you can't afford a hands-free kit?

A prime example of obstruction occurred when I was on an emergency call and attempted to wind my way around the busy London traffic. There were roadworks at the junction of two busy roads and this was causing a long, slow-moving queue of traffic. I had made it as far as a T-junction but was blocked in by a stretch limousine that was straddling the middle of the road, attempting to turn right. Unfortunately, he was himself being blocked by the traffic, which had stopped on the main road running across the junction. I was effectively trapped where I stopped. My lights were on but I switched off my siren; there was little point in keeping it blaring when I was stationary.

The traffic started to move on the main road and the stretch limo tried to clear my path by moving forward and into the flow. This would have solved the problem immediately, and I would have gone on my merry way, arriving only a minute or so late with some luck. However, a coach driver - who had seen and heard me earlier - decided he wasn't going to let the limo driver through and moved forward into the space created by the flow. He effectively blocked the space that the limo driver could have used to free me up. It was the most selfish piece of driving I have seen in a long while.

So now I was blocked again with no hope of getting forward, because the coach was too long to clear the space immediately. The driver just sat in his seat, ignoring me, so I got out of my car and spoke to him through his window.

'You're deliberately obstructing me,' I said. 'Did you not know you can be fined for doing that now?'

I didn't impress him at all and he just ignored me. I looked around, hoping to see a policeman. As I looked back, the coach driver pointed an accusatory finger at the limo driver and shrugged. Disgusting.

'Thanks,' I said.

Funnily enough, and just to confuse matters, drivers can be prosecuted for not obstructing us, too. This story appeared in the *Bury Times*:

A motorist was fined for driving through a red light in Bury after manoeuvring to make space for emergency vehicles.

Steve Whittam was caught on camera driving through a red light at 16mph on Angouleme Way. He made the manoeuvre after pulling to a stop to allow a police van that was using sirens and blue lights to pass him.

He said at a hearing before Bury magistrate on Monday that moving off through the red light after the police van had been the safest thing to do to avoid blocking the path of any further emergency vehicles.

He said: "I was in a dangerous position, stopped across two lanes of very congested traffic. For all I knew there could have been more emergency vehicles on their way. They would not have been able to get through."

He told magistrates during the trial that he admitted driving through the red light but had pleaded not guilty because he thought that was the only way to get an opportunity to explain the circumstances.

The incident happened at the junction with Knowsley Street at about 10.45am on February 13.

Magistrates said they had sympathy with Whittam but saw no special circumstances to excuse his offence. They fined the financial adviser, who lives in Chester, £120 plus £250 costs and put three penalty points on his driving licence.

Mr Whittam (46) told magistrates: "I think it's disgraceful. I did what I thought was the safest thing to help the police and other drivers. I could have just paid the fine and forgotten about it but I wanted to come to court to explain the circumstances as a matter of principle."

Red lights are always a problem. When we drive up behind the car at the front of the queue at traffic lights on red, most drivers will move out of the way. As long as they don't cross too far into the road, that should be fine. But some people simply refuse to move at all. I imagine they're worried they'll be prosecuted for running the light, like Mr Whittam. Surely the fact that they were only doing it for an emergency vehicle should justify the action?

Apparently not. I'm willing to bet that whether or not you earn a ticket for being public-spirited largely depends on the police force and how it views such 'offences', but speaking from my own point of view, I really need drivers to move out of the way, even if that means crossing a red light. If they don't, especially in central London, I could lose two or three minutes of valuable time. Clearly something needs to be done to clear up the law here.

Sirens seem to bug people more and more these days. It's a legal requirement that we use our lights and sirens in order to forewarn you that we are there, and they are a necessary evil. I don't understand why, but I increasingly see people plugging their ears as we approach, and even shouting abuse or shaking their fists at us when we pass, as if we will suddenly stop the noise to appease them.

I was on an emergency call in Soho, where admittedly the narrow streets and closed-in buildings can amplify sound, when I was screamed at by a man who was walking along the pavement. I had my window down so could hear him, but I doubt he would have been silenced if I had wound the window back up.

'Oh, shut up!' he yelled.

I couldn't believe he was directing this at me, and I looked across at him to check. Sure enough, there he was, all purple-faced and angry. How dare I use noise to warn people that I'm coming? From now on, I'll look out for him and ensure that I switch everything off and glide past as I freewheel to my destination.

If he were to drop down in the street with a heart attack any time soon, and found himself hovering between life and death, perhaps he would be a little less keen on the sound of silence.

CREEPY CALLS

Calls in the dead of night can sometimes be unnerving when you're working alone on the FRU. The prospect of going into dark estates and facing threats until back-up arrives is one of the reasons many people in the service prefer not to volunteer for the job. There's a great deal of comfort to be gained from knowing that your crewmate is watching your back; these days nobody in the emergency services is immune to sudden and unprovoked attack.

A FRU paramedic attended a collapsed woman recently and found himself being held hostage in a bed-sit after her husband closed and locked the door and refused to let him out. That situation was only defused when the medic threatened to call the police. In a separate incident, a female responder was threatened with a knife by a gang of youths who approached her car and demanded she give them her stab vest. She, too, escaped harm, staying in the vehicle and calling the police. The gang ran off.

A call to a block of flats in a dodgy part of London made me pause before going in when the woman who answered the intercom sounded threatening towards me. She refused to buzz the door open at first and simply hung up when I told her I was from the ambulance service; a crew was already inside and Control had reported a 'disturbance and raised voices' in the background. I had been asked to be cautious and to report any incident for police backup, and when I eventually got in I found the crew dealing with two noisy drunks and an aggressive female (the one who wouldn't buzz me in). Nothing too serious, as it turned out; it was difficult to make the decision to go into the premises before I knew what was going on, but sometimes instinct works out well.

Then a call to another block of flats in a large estate where one patient, known to be violent, had already threatened a crew that had been there earlier that day. This time the call was to the flat opposite, but every nerve in my body was screaming with preparedness to get the hell out of there if the nutcase from across the corridor decided to come out and have a go. I had to keep watching out for movement behind me as I headed towards the address after stepping out of the lift. To be honest, I had expected him to be at the doors when they opened - I would've had no way of escaping.

A patient who had just been assaulted called the police and ambulance but my crewmate and I were there first, so we went into the address to treat the woman concerned for cuts and bruises. I went out to get the chair for my colleague and heard the front door of the premises slam shut. I turned around to see a man running away from the house and I went back to see what was happening. I got back in to be told that the assailant had been in the house all along. My colleague had been on his own when the guy had appeared from upstairs and decided to leg it. Luckily for him, the man wasn't brave or stupid enough to do anything worse.

Some callers deliberately make life more than a little uncomfortable for us at times. I went to a block of flats in a run-down estate for an *unknown male with chest pain*. The call had come through to us from the police. The details included a statement that the line had 'gone dead' and I was sent to investigate. I went up to the relevant floor of the building and knocked on the door. Nobody answered. I knocked again and again, each time shouting out that I was with the ambulance service. I was greeted by nothing but silence.

I was beginning to wonder about how real this call was. Hoax calls are common in this part of London and I wouldn't be the first paramedic to go knocking on the door of an unwitting person's flat as they tried to sleep after a hard night shift. *I'm going to end up getting a black eye for my trouble here*, I thought.

I persevered, however, because it also wouldn't be the first time that someone had dialled 999 and then promptly died in their own front room.

I pushed on the door and it creaked open. This was starting to feel like something out of a 'B' movie horror film. I cautiously pushed it some more until I could see inside the flat.

'Hello? Anyone there?' I shouted.

Silence. I wasn't feeling safe with this. The flat was small and dingy, and this was a rough neighbourhood. The fact that this person's door was unlocked and set for me to come in on my own was giving me the creeps.

I pushed the door wider and saw a large black guy slumped in an armchair in the front room. He looked about 25 years old, so I was even more concerned about this 'chest pain' call. I stepped inside, calling all the time to see if he would move, but he didn't. I looked left and right to check the rooms either side of me (you never know who might be lurking in the shadows) and continued forward until I got to the man in the chair. He was clearly breathing. He looked asleep but his body was slumped in an unnatural way.

I shook him hard a couple of times and he opened his eyes. He stared right at me and looked as surprised as I felt.

'Did you call an ambulance?' I asked.

'No, I called the police,' he replied, shuffling himself into a more comfortable position.

'You called and said you had chest pain, right?'

'Yeah, but only because the police wouldn't come when I asked them to.'

I wasn't pleased with him, I can tell you. He had been feigning this. It was all an act. When I finally gleaned what had prompted him to call, he told me his flatmate had robbed him.

He had come home to find all he owned gone and had called the police. When they weren't immediately sympathetic, he had decided to add in the fact that he had chest pains - he must have hung up on them for added effect. The police had contacted us and I was sent to check it out - seems all a bit back to front, doesn't it?

The guy had stayed absolutely still while I shouted down the hall at him and worried about my own safety. I'd thought I was walking into a murdered man's flat and that the murderer may well still be there, waiting to knife a cop and getting me instead.

Without wanting to stereotype people, the recent influx of Lithuanians to London has presented us with additional risks. Most of them are hard-working people who cause no bother, but, as with any nationality, some are nasty pieces of work. In my experience, when they drink they can become aggressive. They also tend to be big and unafraid of a punch-up. When they aren't lolling about in a drunken stupor on a bus, they are giving me reason to worry about my personal safety.

A call to a flat in Clapton for a 'man who is bleeding' left me sitting in the ambulance wondering why there was no detail other than that. Why was he bleeding, for example? Where was he bleeding from? How much blood was there?

We entered the housing complex and made our way up a flight of stairs to a badly-maintained and dimly-lit floor containing ten or so flats, the numbering of which was anyone's guess unless you happened to live there.

We found the right place - by accident - and knocked on the door. It was answered by a large, broad man with a thick accent and foul, beery breath. He wanted us to go inside and check his friend out because 'he ish hurrrt'. I wasn't sure about this and neither was my crewmate. The flat had no lights on inside, and we had no way of knowing what the hell was really going on. But he was insistent and, not wanting to be seen as cowards, we crept inside to the hallway.

'You close door now!' he spat.

Not a chance in hell, I thought.

'No, I'd like it to stay open if you don't mind,' I said. 'The light is very bad.'

I was trying diplomacy and giving us an escape route if things went bad. I hoped he was buying it.

'No, no, door must close!'

'No, we won't go any further unless it is open.'

I really must learn Russian. It may not be their first language, but people from the Baltic states all speak Russian as a result of 40-odd years of Soviet occupation.

He gave in and pointed to the room ahead of us. I presumed, correctly, that it was the living room. Another door, to the right, was open and it looked like a bedroom. We walked in to the room ahead after him (neither of us wanted him at our back) and his friend, who was smaller, but only by a notch, was sitting on the sofa with a cut to his hand. It looked, even from a distance, like a knife wound.

'What happened to you?' I asked.

'Cut myself on blade,' he said, his speech quick and garbled.

'Accidentally?'

'Nyes.' I took that as 'Yes'.

'What were you doing when you cut yourself?' I honestly didn't want to know. The lights were still off and I felt very uneasy because my crewmate was looking into the other room, the bedroom with the open door, and the first Lithuanian man was watching him with suspicion.

'Hey!' he shouted. 'What you doing there?'

My crewmate jumped out of the darkness and hurried into the room I was in, with the tall, wide man lurching after him as if he had just stolen the family silver. He had, in fact, been checking to see if there was anybody else in the flat; anyone who could have posed a threat to us.

'Put this light on please,' I said, as firmly as I could.

No-one moved, so I reached for the switch. The man physically tried to stop me from switching it on.

'Look,' I said, slowly and carefully. 'If we don't have the light on, we will leave and your friend won't get any help.'

He backed off and I switched on the main light to the front room. My crewmate was back in the hallway, peering back into the bedroom. This time he had the leaking light to help him see.

I was in mid-sentence with the man with the injured hand when my colleague came up to me and said, quietly, 'I'm getting out of here.'

That got the hairs on the back of my neck standing up in a flash. *What the hell is going on?*

I tried to follow because 'I'm getting out of here' is code for 'Let's both of us get the f**k out of here now'. But my way was barred by the broad man, and now he had attitude.

'Where he goink?' he shouted, in my face.

'He's leaving and I need to go with him because we need to discuss the patient,' I lied.

He put his massive paw on my shoulder and attempted to sit me down next to his sorry, bleeding flatmate, but I resisted and pushed it aside, trying to keep my balance at the same time.

'No, you stay and help my friend.'

'I will help him,' I said, 'but only if you calm down and get out of my way so that I can leave for a few moments.'

A few seconds of nervous tension passed as we stared at each other. I never once let this guy out of my sight. This wasn't going well, and I felt in imminent danger. I didn't have my stab vest on and I knew there was a knife around somewhere. I might be in serious trouble if I didn't negotiate my way out of here.

'Look, I'll come back and deal with your friend,' I said. 'But you have both been aggressive and my colleague has left for his safety and I should leave too.'

I think he was confused by this. I think he wondered why we felt intimidated by their behaviour, especially his behaviour. He moved out of my way and I picked up my bags and left the flat.

When I got back to the ambulance my crewmate had already alerted the police and a Duty Officer.

'What the hell was that all about?' I asked him.

'There was blood all over the walls of that bedroom,' he said. 'It looks like somebody has been murdered in there.'

We waited until the cops arrived and told them what had happened before our hasty exit. We watched them go up in force and thump on the door.

'Police. Open up!'

Nothing. Not a sound.

They thumped on the door again, much harder this time, and the neighbours began to appear at their windows and doors.

'Police. Open this door now!'

They didn't reply. We both watched and wondered what was going to happen next.

After three or four more attempts, the police broke down the door and charged inside. We saw one of them struggle with the wide Lithuanian man. Then it all went quiet. They spent no more than ten minutes inside before re-appearing. One of the officers came up to us and told us that the man with the cut hand had been trying to hurt himself in a drunken rage earlier and the blood on the walls was the result of him smearing it all over the bedroom after he had cut his hand open. It was a bizarre but strangely credible explanation, though their threatening behaviour inside that dark, little dump they called home had still been unacceptable.

Night-time psychiatric calls have their own potential. One night, when we were particularly busy and the police were run off their feet, my crewmate and I were called to an address for a violent man with mental health problems - he was a schizophrenic. We were warned to wait until police arrived because he had already assaulted someone and was known to use weapons. We parked up at the end of the road out of sight and waited for backup to arrive, but a figure on the street started to move towards us, shouting and waving his arms frantically. I told my crewmate that I thought this might be our man and that we had been spotted. We watched as he drew closer and I started the engine of the ambulance for a quick exit if needed; he held his ground in the middle of the road and now we had no way out.

He stood there, shouting and gesticulating in a very threatening manner, and we called for an ETA on the police. There were no units available so we had to sit this out. He carried on his erratic behaviour and began to get closer to the vehicle again.

Just as we were preparing to leave by whatever means we could, a lone police officer arrived in a patrol car. He immediately approached the man and a struggle broke out, with the cop trying to wrestle him to the ground. We got out and helped bring him under control, and he was cuffed by the officer before he became any more of a threat. Luckily, he had no weapons because I'm sure he would have used them.

We sat there, the four of us, sweating and shaking with adrenaline, sucking in lungfuls of air. I looked at the policeman; he wasn't huge and he didn't look all that tough, but how brave was he?

I have transferred a couple of psychiatric patients that have a place in my memory. One of them was a young girl who had murdered her sister and was being taken from one secure unit to another. A nurse escort was provided and in these cases they tend to be very large men, which is comforting. For some reason, this girl was intent on psyching me out and stared relentlessly at me in the rear view mirror as I drove the ambulance. Every time I looked into it to check the back I saw her eyes burning into me - they never wavered, not once. Thoughts of Jack Nicholson's face through that broken door in *The Shining* ran through my head.

Worse was to come. The girl demanded cigarettes and the psychiatric nurse decided to buy her some to keep her quiet. He asked us to stop while he got out of the vehicle and went to get them from a little shop. This was not an emergency transfer, so a stop like this wasn't out of protocol, but it left me and my crewmate alone with her. She continued to stare at me and, in a hushed tone reminiscent of every horror movie murderer you've ever heard, said, 'I stabbed my sister, you know.'

Yeah, I knew. I knew twice now, and I wanted that nurse back pronto.

On the subject of murdered sisters, another patient who was being transferred while I was 'third manning' (a crew plus me) repeatedly demanded to know who had killed her mother. She had murdered her own sister and was convinced that someone else had killed her mother, too. She continually barked, 'Who killed my mother, who did it?' as we drove her to hospital. When we arrived and she was being taken into the psychiatric ward, she asked again, very loudly, 'Who killed my mother?' I was walking behind the crew and they thought it might be funny to turn in unison and point directly at me.

Luckily, she didn't see them and I got away with it (their joke, not the murder). Only two of the three of us were smiling about it, though.

Not all calls are creepy because of the potential for harm. Some are just weird and leave you with an uncomfortable feeling afterwards.

I went to the aid of a man who was complaining of chest pain and when I got to his flat I discovered a collection of what I can only describe as sexual torture instruments strewn about the place. I started talking to him as he sat on his sofa and, although his name was Sam, he insisted I call him 'Samantha'. I could clearly see his Adam's apple bobbing up and down and his voice was a couple of octaves down from a woman's. But I thought, *Fair enough, Samantha, if that's how you want it.* It didn't feel right calling him by that name, though.

When the crew arrived, one of them started to take the equipment brought from the ambulance back as 'Samantha' didn't want to go to hospital and was simply emotional. As I spoke to him, I noticed that his gaze had drifted to something in the background. I looked up just in time to see my colleague walking out with a long blonde wig attached by a strand to the Velcro of one of the bags. It looked like a fair-haired puppy was walking behind him. He had no idea.

On the way out of the flat I noticed that 'Samantha' had left photos of himself in suggestive poses and completely naked on the table. They were arranged almost as if he had deliberately laid them out for us to see. Took me a while to get that one out of my head.

* * * * *

Every so often, a shift will start in such a way as to put you on edge, but rarely does a single shift contain such a bizarre chain of events that it is guaranteed to make you re-consider your profession.

Night shift. I was sent into a north London estate to investigate a 999 call made by a resident who claimed that a 14-year-old girl was lying on the road, *'screaming'*. The caller also stated that there was a gang of under-age drinkers hovering around.

I went to the call expecting to see a drunken teenage girl with nothing better to do than draw attention to herself, but when I got on scene there was nobody around. I drove along the street and, as I passed one of the estate complexes, I saw a little gang of teenagers staring at me from a balcony – they all had bottles in their hands.

I decided to stop and ask them if they knew anything about the screaming girl, but before I could pull up I heard a yell, directed at me I think, and then a sudden, loud bang. I thought something had hit the car, so I moved forward to get away from the immediate area. As I did so, I heard the crunch of glass beneath my wheels. The yobs had thrown a glass beer bottle at the vehicle. Luckily it hadn't made contact but had landed on the road in front of it instead. I got clear and called for urgent police assistance.

A few seconds after I called for help, the ambulance crew arrived. Unsuspectingly, they drew up where I had been before, right across from the gang of louts on the balcony. I flashed my headlights at the ambulance and they saw me. They were just about to get out, I think, but instead drove on to where I was, a hundred yards or so away.

When they joined me, I explained what had happened. They had seen the group of young boys and girls on the balcony and hadn't liked the look of them either.

We waited for the police but when they finally arrived most of the gang had gone. We followed the officers up into the complex and found a few of them hanging around trying to look innocent. The police challenged them about what had happened but they denied everything, of course.

'This is harassment,' a scrawny, spotty boy asked. 'Did any of you see me throw a bottle?'

Of course I hadn't seen who had thrown it, I just heard it fall and break in front of me. The glass was still on the road.

The youths continued to deny everything and got a little heated at times about 'harassment' and 'breach of human rights'. They get all that stuff from the TV – modern kids know more about the law than the police, I think.

They were given a warning and we left the scene. I went back to my station and waited for my next call. I was edgy after that little bit of nonsense, so I was glad to get a couple of routine jobs. Then I received a call in south London; it was amber, so not a priority, but it was still a long way to drive, so I called my Control and asked if I was the nearest vehicle. They said I was, and that there were no ambulances assigned, as yet.

When I looked at the call description, it read *'50 year-old male ?# arm'* – I was going to someone who may have broken his arm. Fine. Except, underneath it read *'blood all over chest, ? cause'*, and that worried me. It worried me because it didn't make sense. People with broken arms generally don't have blood all over their chest. Something was wrong with this call, but I was running on it and I waited until I got on scene until I queried it further.

I arrived to find myself driving into a dead end street, deep inside a rough housing estate. It was dark and very quiet and more than a few things were beginning to rattle me. Starting with that call description. I picked up the radio and requested some information.

'I'm on scene,' I said, 'but before I go into the address can you tell me what the caller said about blood being all over the patient's chest?'

'Sorry, he just said that and hung up to go back to the address and wait.'

'In that case, I'm going into this with caution.'

I should have asked about police back-up – I normally would – but tonight there just seemed to be nobody around to help. The police hadn't arrived for 15 minutes on the broken bottle call so there was little chance of a speedy response to this one, especially as all I had was a bad feeling.

A car drew up across from me and its headlights shone on me as I got my bags from the car. The driver seemed overly-interested in me and I kept an eye on him. A woman stood outside a pub on the corner. It was late into the night, around 2am, so I figured she must be the landlady. She just stared at me, too. It was all becoming a little more than unsettling now.

The flat I needed to reach was on the first floor and there was scaffolding all around the building, so once I was up there I wouldn't be visible from the street. I considered waiting until the ambulance crew arrived but I called myself a coward in my head and went to do my job.

I climbed the steps leading to the first floor very cautiously – a lot more slowly than I normally would have. There wasn't a sound. Every shadow could have been a threat, but nothing moved. The guy in the car was still hanging around. I was being watched as I made my way to the address.

Once on the landing, I approached the door of the flat and stood outside for a few seconds. It was one of those flats that you can see into through a couple of small windows at the side of the front door, so I made use of one of them by peering in to see if there was anything amiss. The window looked into the kitchen and I could it was a mess, but that's not unusual in these places. I also saw something else, however, and it rang alarm bells with me. The cutlery drawer was lying open. I should have stopped there and then but instead I looked through the other window and saw that the front room was also a mess. There seemed to be nobody around.

I resolved to knock on the door and watch who came to answer it. If I didn't like the look of the person I would leave the scene and wait for back-up. I stood away from the door and saw an old black man approach to open the door. I felt a little less insecure.

He waved me inside and motioned to the front room.

'He's in there,' he said. 'He's a mess. Help him.' He didn't look at me as he spoke.

I walked into the room, and it looked like an abbatoir. There was blood smeared on every wall. Every piece of furniture had been smashed, as had the television. Something very bad had happened here.

On the sofa to my right sat a tall black man – he, too, was elderly, in his mid 60s at least I thought. He was *covered* in blood and had clear wounds to his head and left arm. They were stab wounds. He had been viciously attacked and it had happened right here and not long ago.

'Is there *anyone* else in this flat?' I asked. I was urgent about this, because I had no idea how much danger I might be in.

'No, only us,' the old man said.

'I'll ask again. Is there anyone else in this flat?'

'No,' they both said.

I looked at the man on the sofa. Some of his wounds were very deep. I saw he had a lethal-looking injury to his throat and penetrating slashes to his skull. He was lucky to be breathing, never mind talking to me.

'I'm in pain,' he moaned. 'My arm is so bad.'

He was cradling an obviously broken left arm. It had either been stabbed so deeply that a bone had broken, or he had been beaten mercilessly. He was still sitting upright, but he was nervy and I still felt uneasy about the company I was in, regardless of their ages.

I dressed the worst wounds at the back of his head. Someone had carved a cross into it. They must have sat on him and done this, because I can't imagine he'd have allowed it to happen without putting up a serious struggle – it must have hurt a lot.

I called my Control and requested urgent police and an ambulance and explained that the situation was not as given. I was stressed and I made it clear on the phone that I wasn't happy.

After a few minutes, the older man answered a knock at the door. I thought a crew had arrived, but instead he let in a man who walked directly towards me.

'Who is this?' I asked.

'He's OK,' the old man said. 'He's a friend.'

'I don't care who he is, he's not coming in here,' I said. 'He needs to go into the bedroom out of the way.'

The situation was getting out of control and I didn't want anyone else in there. I made it clear to both of them and I think they understood.

The crew arrived within ten minutes and they were just as shocked by the scene as I had been. We quickly removed the patient to the safety of the ambulance and began his treatment in earnest. All the while, he denied any knowledge of what had taken place; he seemed deliberately evasive about our questions.

I showed the police into the flat and the scene was sealed for forensics to go over it. I left with the crew and took our patient to the nearest hospital. He wasn't dying, but he had suffered major injuries and we had no idea what kind of internal damage had been done.

After handing the patient over to the hospital staff I was told that he had a history of violence against the police. He had allegedly thrown acid over an officer's face, so he wasn't innocent. I also learned that a bent carving knife had been found in the kitchen sink.

Later that night, rattled as I was, I was sent to a call that seemed routine – a collapsed drunken male. I arrived on scene, where a crew were already dealing with him. His friends were standing around outside the ambulance with the police and I went inside to check if I was needed. I spent five minutes with the crew and left. Everyone had gone from outside and all was quiet.

I jumped into my car and had driven maybe fifty yards up the road when I pulled over to fill in my paperwork for the call. I put my reading light on and was busily filling in the form when I heard a thump from behind me. I recognised the sound of my paramedic bag falling forward – it does that a lot when I'm driving. I glanced over my left shoulder and there, sitting in the darkness of the back seat, were two men. They were just looking at me. I almost jumped out of my skin.

'Who the hell are you two?' I shouted.

They just stared. I thought one of them was going to reach for something; my mind told me it was a weapon.

'What are you doing in this car?' I said.

Then one of them piped up.

'The police officer said to sit in here and wait.'

It turns out they were the drunken man's friends. I threw them both out of the car and they walked off into the distance. I think I sat with my head in my hands for ten minutes after that. Funny thing, paranoia.

* * * * *

Other creepy calls are menacing because they set up atmospheres of potential threat even before you get on scene. Most of the time, the police are present or they have been called and we are advised to sit tight until they appear, but sometimes you walk straight into a situation without pre-warning and where the police are present but powerless to cover your back.

A domestic assault call in east London took me and my crewmate out of area in the middle of the night to help a teenage mum who had allegedly been beaten up and threatened with a knife by her boyfriend. He had cut her across the face and given her more than a few bumps and bruises around the head as he laid into her with fists and feet - all because she wouldn't let him go out with his mates. A nice guy, then.

As if proof of that were needed, he had recently come out of prison, where he had served a sentence for grievous bodily harm. The police, who were on scene, suspected he was still lurking around outside but hadn't the personnel to go searching for him.

I had to leave the house to get equipment from the ambulance while my crewmate examined and treated the girl. It was dark and very quiet. The house looked onto the back of woodland, so there was no light to move by. I wished the cops hadn't told me he was lurking around out here because now it felt like every tree was watching me. I almost expected him to pounce on me at any second. As far as I was aware, he wasn't armed - the knife had been left at home when he ran off - but that was of little comfort to me as I rooted around inside the ambulance at three in the morning, knowing that I had to get back out and that, somewhere in the shadows, this guy might be following my every move. I doubted the security that the presence of a single police vehicle gave me, so I was very cautious when I jumped down from the vehicle. We had no torch on board, so all I had was my keen eyesight - next to useless in this pitch blackness. I got out, equipment in hand (none of which would be useful as a weapon), and peered around into the dark and then up towards the house itself. Nothing stirred. All I could hear was the sound of a few trees creaking in the cold breeze. The only light visible was the one coming from the patient's kitchen window.

I crept back towards that light with my eyes focusing on anything that looked remotely human in shape. Then... damn it. I realised I hadn't locked the ambulance. I couldn't risk this psychopath getting into the back of it and lying in wait for us when we brought his girlfriend out. There was no remote lock on the vehicle; it had to be done manually. I had to go back.

I returned as cautiously as I had left and fumbled the key into the door lock as I looked around and listened. The lock engaged and I checked the door - it was secure.

Then there was a sudden crashing noise behind me. I froze. I could hear scrabbling, as if someone was running from the woods, and a shape darted across my field of vision. I held my breath. Then I picked up the shape of the running thing. It was small and dark and fat.

Bloody cat.

THE FESTIVE SEASON

During the Christmas period, which can start as early as the first of October depending on how needy or juvenile you are, there is a measurable increase in the consumption of alcohol. It's measurable and it's different because the calls we receive include those from professionals, City types and 'normal' people - the kind of person we don't see much of during the rest of the year. It seems as though, for some, the office Christmas party is a real good excuse to get off your face and tell your boss what you think of him. The trouble is, I am often mistaken for their boss and so I receive the venom.

I went to a call at an underground station near Oxford Street for a woman who had fallen over and cut her head. When I went into the staff office I could see that she was drunk. She was also belligerent. I tried to be nice to her but no amount of Mr Nice Guy would shut her up. She insulted me, stared at me with drunken glassy eyes and tried to claw at me when I attempted to check her blood sugar.

This woman was with her new boss, and he was drunk too. He wasn't drunk enough to escape feeling embarrassed, though; he apologised again and again while trying to reason with this obnoxious woman. She wasn't to be reasoned with, however; I got the feeling she was unreasonable by nature, and that drink just uncorked the personality she kept tightly bottled up most of the time.

Eventually, with her clawing and scratching, she managed to cut my hand. I wasn't happy with that. 'I'm not treating you any more,' I said, raising my voice and showing her the marks she had left.

'Fine,' she yelled. 'I don't want your f**king treatment anyway!'

'Fine,' I replied. 'But you have a cut to the head and you're drunk, so you need to be taken home.'

'How dare you speak to me like that!'

I think she was offended by my tone, but I was beyond caring. She represented the worst kind of drunk to me; there are honest drunks, who can happily get on with it and admit they need help, and then there are the others - dishonest drunks, with hidden problems. This kind of drunk spits and whines in the face of all those who are willing and able to offer a helping hand. This kind of drunk berates the ambulance service or the police service or whoever crosses their path in uniform. This kind of drunk uses alcohol to hide their daytime façade and too many glasses of wine exposes their true self.

This kind of drunk wakes up in the morning and thinks, *My God, what did I do?*

Another rude drunk crossed swords with me at a wine bar near Holborn. She had fallen onto the slate floor and cracked her head open. She'd bled quite a bit, but now it was under control. However, her wound would have to be closed properly at hospital.

'I'm going to have to get an ambulance here,' I said.

She flatly refused and instead gave me that silly, drunken stare that smashed people give sober ones - you know, the one that doesn't quite focus and the head begins to drop, so that the eyes are forced up to keep track of their 'victim'. I find it amusing and can't help smiling when they do it. This, of course, gets me penalty points and a barrage of verbal abuse for being a 'smarmy git'.

Her friend, a tall, well-built and equally drunk man, took me aside.

'Look, mate,' he said. 'Between you and me, don't tell anyone, we're both police officers. I mean, she's a bit lary at the moment but she's basically a good girl.'

I nodded.

'Plus we're not really supposed to be out together. If you know what I mean.'

'Well, that's interesting,' I said, 'but it's not really relevant to me. She needs to go to hospital and get that head fixed, or else it's going to get infected and cause all sorts of bigger problems.'

He nodded. She just became more and more abusive.

'I'm not going to hospital,' she shouted. 'I've f**king told you once. Or twice? I dunno, but I've told you. So you can f**k off and take your little ambulance car with you.'

She pointed out of the doorway to the FRU car. I felt slighted by this remark. Really, I did.

She tore off the dressing and bandage that I had just carefully placed on her head and threw it to the floor. It was stained red with her blood.

'Look,' I said. 'I strongly advise you to go and get that wound treated. It will get infected or might re-open again later on.'

'I'm not going anywhere and that's that. Why don't you leave me alone?'

The guy with her stepped between us and tried to persuade her to calm down, and she erupted in his face. I think there was more than a little tension between them.

I stood back and watched the fireworks until a crew arrived. I explained the situation to them and they continued to try and get her to go to hospital. The police had also arrived by now, because the ruckus she was causing had forced the bar owner to call them in. Another whispered exchange took place between the tall man and the police officers, and somehow the screaming, uncooperative woman was persuaded to go to the ambulance and get checked out. At least then she could calm down and comply - or refuse and sign the appropriate form (if you refuse to go to hospital you will be asked to sign our PRF).

I left the scene before she decided to get going on her second wind. So much for trying to help.

> **PRF. Patient Report Form. A cumbersome three-part, carbon-backed form used to record absolutely every detail of a call. It can be used as a legal document in court.**

There are otherwise perfectly decent types who get drunk and then have no idea how to limit their excesses. This can lead to serious injury which could have a life-long effect, so I would think that once you've sobered up with your damaged brain and the threat of permanent episodes of epilepsy, you would consider your actions and how they have ruined you life. What I don't know is how many of these people resolve never to drink so irresponsibly again, and how many end up in hospital every Christmas.

A seasonal call to the City for a man who had fallen down the steps at an underground station. He had toppled head-long down ten or so concrete steps and landed, unconscious, at the bottom, much to the disgust of his fellow commuters, most of whom had looked, tutted and marched off home or wherever they usually marched off to.

I arrived to find him slumped against the wall, where the Underground staff had propped him. Around about then, he regained consciousness and attempted to get up and walk. He had a severe head injury and was probably the most drunken person in a suit I have ever seen. He looked like a banker.

This guy was over 6ft tall, wide-shouldered and looked more than capable of taking care of himself - except when he drank. Now he couldn't even walk.

He groaned and moaned about the state of his head, which had been bleeding badly but was now under control. He told passing commuters (some of whom were still tutting) to 'p*ss off' and he was generally unpleasant. Except to me. He was very nice to me and even thanked me for being there for him, which made a change.

I explained that he had fallen down the steps and now needed to go to hospital, but he was insistent that he could get home.

'I'm OK now, thanks,' he said, his voice slow and slurred. 'I'm happy to take a taxi home'.

'I don't think any taxi will be happy to take you, though,' I said.

'Am I drunk?'

'Yes, you are. You are very drunk.'

'Did I fall?'

'Yes. Down those steps. I told you earlier.'

'Did you? Why did I fall?'

'Because you're drunk.'

'Am I drunk?'

The conversation cycled like that for five or six minutes while I waited for an ambulance to rescue me from it. The man was clearly concussed and I briefly handed over to the London Underground guy, letting him answer the same questions for a couple of cycles. It was highly amusing to watch - he looked like he was teaching a teddy bear the times tables.

'Yes... you... fell... and... hit... your... head.'

'Why?'

'Because... you... drank... too... much.'

'Oh… am I drunk?'

Ad almost infinitum.

Christmas is but the start of it all; however; the real fun begins at the *end* of the year.

New Year's Eve is unique in the ambulance service calendar. Virtually all of our resources are deployed, and we're still pushed to the limit. The voluntary services are roped in to help *en masse* - many of them are based at our stations for the night - and there are first aid centres opened up all over the place. We aren't the only emergency service out in force; the police and fire services are also at full capacity in terms of manpower and equipment. Overtime is offered to all those not normally rostered to work on that date, and there are officers all over the place, some of whom have rarely seen the light of day since last New Year.

On December 31 we deal with more alcohol-related calls than any other day of the year. Habitual drunks love this time of year, because they can get absolutely smashed and for once they will actually blend in with the rest of society. Ordinary people down as much cider or beer or wine as their stomach can contain in a race to beat the bells, almost as if it's some sort of crime not to be as drunk as a skunk before midnight comes.

The only sober people around are the people doing the hard work, the public servants who are on duty, the bar and night club staff, the taxi, bus and tube drivers. Everyone else, including the kids in some cases, gets hammered from the moment they touch the gold-paved streets of central London.

Last New Year's Eve was much like any other. I was busy that night, of course, as was everyone else on duty. The calls were coming in thick and fast, even before the hour of midnight struck; after that, it went crazy, and it was relentless and extremely exhausting. I had been stuck in heavy traffic just after the bells, and thousands of people were filling the roads. I couldn't move the car at all for about twenty minutes and call after call came in to me, only to be cancelled at my request because I just couldn't take them.

Then I got called (when finally free of the human soup) to a *'non-responsive man in street'* and ended up being flagged down by the police in Whitehall where a guy had collapsed right next to Downing Street. I can tell you right now they get very nervous about that sort of thing. They don't like it when you fall down so close to the seat of Government. The man could have been a terrorist. Or a Conservative.

He wasn't. He was just another drunk - a tall, thin drunk with an equally tall, equally thin mate who continually apologised about the state of his friend, who was now vomiting all over the pavement as if he had an endless supply of the stuff in his stomach and secreted elsewhere around his body. I am often surprised by the volume of sick some people can emit; it seems to exceed the capacity of their insides, as though they have become some sort of vomitary human Tardis.

So I waited with him, and I waited and waited. No ambulances were available. The crews were all running around London, saving lives and livers. I was waiting because I had no hope of getting a vehicle. The armed police guarding Downing Street were getting more interested in us than usual and a couple of officers sidled up to enquire as to how long we thought we'd be and what exactly was going on.

I needed a plan. As I considered my options, a solution crossed my line of sight; a voluntary services bod with an empty trolley bed. Why he was wheeling it up Whitehall was beyond me, but it was the answer I needed. I commandeered him and his trolley bed (it turns out he was delivering it back on foot to the treatment centre up the road) and explained my situation.

We loaded the drunk onto the bed and wheeled him up the middle of Whitehall to the sanctuary of what I hoped would be an accommodating treatment vehicle owned by the St John Ambulance. No such luck. They wouldn't have him. They had two in there already. I was seriously considering lying him down on the back seat of the car and driving him to hospital myself when a Service Patient Transport vehicle arrived.

'Can you take this bloke?' I asked, my spirits rising.

Unfortunately, the St J A had other ideas; they wanted this vehicle too. I thought I was going to be stuck with this vomiting man all morning when some ambulance officers showed up and changed the plan. Soon enough he was off my hands and on his way to infamy (when he got home).

That call was followed by another drunk, this time at Victoria station - a young girl. Her friends said she was 23 but she and they looked more like 13 to me and the cops who were there. Again, no ambulance available, so it looked like I was stuck with her for the foreseeable future. She wasn't in serious danger; the worst that was going to happen to her was that she would sober up and have a hangover, and maybe learn a lesson. But I couldn't just leave her because I believed that she was a minor. Drunk minors have to go somewhere, to a place of safety, and if I was right with my guesstimate and I walked away from her then I would be in real trouble.

She was lying on the ground and getting colder, despite my blankets and warm reassurances. An audience of queuing fast-foodies were watching with docile, cow-like interest. One or two shouted out sexual innuendos, and others yelled snide remarks at the police. Imaginative stuff, like 'Don't you have anything better to do?' Catching sight of my grim face, one of them said, 'Cheer up, mate, it's New Year's Eve.' Thing is, I look grim because I'm not happy, and I'm not happy because I've got better and, frankly, more important things to be doing.

In the end, I bundled her and an attending WPC into the back of my car and drove them to the nearest hospital, hoping she would behave and not throw up all over the back seat because I was going to have more 'patients' to convey before the night was done.

* * * * *

Let's not forget the other activity that is rife during the Christmas and New Year celebrations - violence.

It may be the season to be jolly and all that, but for many it's the ideal time to dust off the knives, guns and baseball bats and get to work. There were almost 40 stabbings in London during the festivities last year, and across the country a large number of violent crimes were recorded. One woman, a young bar owner and a mother of two, died after trying to break up a scuffle in her pub just before closing time. She was knocked to the floor and rendered unconscious and she never woke up. See, that's the reality of pub fights. They're dirty and nasty and mean and they sometimes claim lives. Whoever knocked that woman over didn't know about her two kids and didn't mean to kill her. They were just fighting drunk and out of control; but the result was a massive human tragedy that put terrible holes in other people's lives.

Drugs also play a big part in the festivities. For some reason, and probably the same one that the drunks use, drug addicts and abusers tend to increase their consumption of whatever they can get hold of on the last day of the old year.

My final call came in five minutes before I ended my shift. Usually you're left alone until you finish for the last 20 minutes or so, but not this time. The call was for a 23 year old man having an *'art attack'*. I had to get on the phone to the FRU desk about this one.

'Hello,' I said. 'Have you actually read the description for this call?'

'Erm, no,' the controller said. 'Let me have a look.'

Short pause.

'Oh, yeah. I see what you mean. Sorry. Still, he needs to be checked out. Do you mind?'

'Not at all. Pleasure,' I replied. It was almost 7am, I was knackered and in a sarcastic mood, to be honest.

I drove to the location and landed up in a sleazy alleyway near London Bridge. I kept my eyes peeled but I didn't get out of the vehicle because I was uneasy about this. I couldn't see anyone; it looked like a hoax or as though the caller had simply left after waiting a fairly long time. But as I turned the car around to go, I spotted a hooded youth sitting on the wall across from me. He was staring at me and I guessed he might be the caller. I didn't like the look of him and decided to stay in the car and roll down the window.

'Hello?' I called. 'Did you call an ambulance?'

'Yeah,' he mumbled. 'I'm out of it and I think my heart is going to stop. I think I might be 'avin an 'art attack.'

A little light went on in my head.

I sized him up, decided I could cope with him if it turned nasty, and got out of the car. I tried to look as big as possible, breathing deeply and squaring my shoulders.

'What have you been taking tonight?'

'Ecstasy and other sh*t. My heart's goin' really fast. I'm dyin'.'

I assumed he was exaggerating, but I checked his pulse and other obs, anyway. He had a fast heart beat, sure enough, but nothing critical was going on with him, he was just clucking a bit.

TACHYCARDIA. A fast heart rate. A heart rate above 100 beats per minute in adults is considered tachycardic. Sometimes the word is shortened to 'tachy', as in 'the patient was tachy at 130'. As distinct from 'Bradycardia', a slow heart rate. In adults this term is applied when the HR is less than 60 bpm. In athletes and other individuals it may be perfectly normal to have such a low heart rate, however, and the term is only applied clinically where the rate is seen as abnormal for the patient.

I weighed up the options. He looked evil: he just had one of those faces, dangerous and mean, and he was also out of his skull. Very hyper, very edgy and very unpredictable. We aren't allowed to search people - the best I can do is say to them, 'Do you have anything on you that will harm you or me?' If the police are there you can ask them to perform a search, but otherwise you have to take people at their word. I was uncomfortable with the thought of having to take him to hospital myself. As he sat in the back of the car, my head and neck would be very exposed to him. But I wouldn't get an ambulance at this time on this day - and I'd have considered it a waste of resources, anyway. The police were too busy to help. I wanted to go home. But I couldn't leave him here. It was a conundrum with only one solution.

Much as I didn't want to, I was going to have to take him. 'OK,' I said. 'In you get.'

He climbed in and when he finally strapped himself in - I had to tell him twice - I started up and drove off. Instantly, he wanted to be my mate. That always makes me suspicious, straight away. When people are leaning over a lot, and getting really close to you to talk to you, behaving like they've known you for years, I don't like it. It sets alarm bells ringing.

'Those bastards,' he said. 'They stitched me up.'

I said nothing, but just nodded, not wanting to get involved in conversation.

He sat back and started ranting. From what I could make out, he'd gone out for the night with a mate and his mate had dumped him. To make matters worse, they had gone out for drugs and he'd only got half of what he had paid for. He alternated between shouting and mumbling, and gradually he started directing the shouting at me. He sounded like he was ready to pop at any moment, as though I was his enemy rather than someone who was trying to help him.

He turned from his traitorous friend to the medical staff awaiting him at hospital. 'What are they going to do to me?' he yelled. 'They're just going to kick me out, aren't they?'

I glanced into that rear-view mirror more times than I ought to have done, considering I was driving, and I had my foot as close to the floor as I could safely get it. But the streets were now clear and we eventually got to our destination without him making any moves on me.

I left him sitting in the reception area of the hospital. They wouldn't take him in any of the wards because they were full and he wasn't an emergency. Neither were many of the residents of the cubicles, to be honest, but once you have a bed, you're home and dry. As far as New Year's Eve goes... them's the rules.

HORRIBLE HOUSING

There are some parts of London which you would never venture into at night unless you had to.

Unfortunately, we do have to. We're wary when the calls come in. Often, it's not only that these places are dangerous, but that some of them are so badly-designed that getting into them, whether safely or not, is a navigational nightmare (this is true at any time of the day, it's just harder to find your way around at night).

The old London County Council estates are some of the largest in Europe and contain some of the worst construction designs I have ever seen. Lloyd George's Housing Act of 1919, where the pledge of 'homes for heroes' seemed to promise a new dawn in architectural excellence, instead produced examples of poorly-planned construction that still exist today. The people now housed in these estates are the immigrants, the elderly and the poorest of society. In some ways, they are heroes just for putting up with it.

One word that always makes me cringe when I see it on the screen is 'Peabody'. The Peabody Donation Fund was set up in 1852 by an American banker called George Peabody. He'd done well out of life and yet he was troubled by the poverty and misery he saw all around him. Rather nobly, he decided to do something about it and set up a fund to provide housing for the city's poor. The Trust that bears his name now owns or manages over 19,000 properties and houses almost 50,000 people across London.

So far, so good. Unfortunately, what was an improvement over the conditions which had previously characterised Victorian England is not - in my opinion - suitable for a crowded, modern city of eight or nine million. It's not the ugliness of these places, and they *are* ugly: I'm not a commentator on architectural design, but I know an eyesore when I see one and I know a badly-designed pile of bricks when I go *into* one. No, the ugliness of some of these estates is not an issue for me, because I don't have to live in them, thank goodness. What annoys me is the difficulty in getting access to them when you are responding to an emergency call.

You try finding a gasping, dying man in a top floor flat on one of the Peabody estates - or any of the capital's tower blocks and rabbit runs - at 4am on a dark, rainy November morning, when half the lights aren't working and the lift is bust (or non-existent). It's not easy, and we're in a profession where lost minutes - lost seconds, even - can mean the difference between life and death.

Sometimes, it's almost as though whoever built these places deliberately put obstacles in the way of the emergency services: numbering that makes no sense, stairwells that are too narrow or in odd places, bollards placed across roads... it all feels like a conspiracy to stop you getting to the address in question with enough time to do much good for the caller. Many buildings have large gates at the entrance to the car park. Yes, people need to feel secure, and a good, solid gate with a strong lock will help, but if an ambulance crew has to stand at it for 10 minutes until somebody finds the key or remembers the access code, then from time to time this will cost a life. We do get given keys ourselves, but there are so many of them, and it only takes someone to lose a bunch, or have them stolen, and you're in serious trouble. (A better system, and one used by many old people's homes, is coded entry: these numbers are held centrally and sent to us via our screens as and when needed.)

On most estates, the blocks all look absolutely identical with only a small identifying name plate to help you distinguish one from another. These are rarely well-lit and finding and reading them is a task and a half. It's bad enough when you're in an ambulance, with a crewmate to look whilst you drive, but on the FRU you are driving and looking at the same time and it's next to impossible.

This all compounds the stress you feel when you head to a call you already know is serious, one where you need to be with the patient very quickly. Standing outside in the rain looking up at an illegible map on a graffiti-covered map-board is *not* helpful. Even a routine call can quickly turn tragic.

I was sent to a 72-year-old man who was suffering difficulty in breathing (DIB). I sped to the estate and found myself, once again, trying to see the map and locate the relevant building. I saw that it was on the opposite side to where I had stopped and realised it would take a few minutes to walk round. Then I saw the ambulance appear on that side and decided to drive round and join the crew; *They obviously knew the place better than me*, I thought.

I got to the other side of the estate and found that my optimism had been misplaced. The ambulance was now reversing out of the car park - it was full, and the driver's only other option would have been a very tight three-point turn. She and her crewmate looked as lost and bewildered as me. There was no visible access to any of the buildings from where we were, and no signs or boards designating each block. They didn't know where to go either.

I was just about to call Control and ask them for a better location, when two young boys appeared, running and waving at me. They pointed to the block of flats just behind them and I hurried over to the ambulance to let the crew know we were at the right spot after all.

I asked one of the boys to take me to the address whilst the other stayed behind to guide the crew in after they had unloaded their bags. I followed him as he unlocked a gate and ran up the path to the block. He then took me up a flight of stairs.

'It's just up here,' he told me as he glanced back.

'Great,' I said. I was carrying all my bags, which must weigh at least 15 kilos. You can add to that the crash bag that I carry, which is another couple of kilos, and then the oxygen, which will be a further couple of kilos. So the fact that we were nearly there was music to my ears. One flight of stairs was enough. (If you're in the business, you already know how this turns out so feel free to skip the next paragraph.)

The first flight led on to the next flight, then another, and then another. I was gasping for air by the time we reached the fourth floor, and I consider myself to be fit. It seemed like an eternity getting up those stairs, laden as I was with the equipment I needed. Where the *hell* was the lift?

Eventually, we got to the door. A huge pile of shoes lay outside. We went into a flat that was heaving with people. They were immigrants, and there tend to be many more of them crammed into one place, usually all from the same family. The shoes are the first hint you get.

The old man was lying in bed, surrounded by seriously-worried family members. He didn't look right - in fact, he was virtually unconscious - and I could see him labouring to breathe. I quickly cleared the room of most of the people, until just the older members of the family and the paramedic from the ambulance were with me.

There was no response from the man, and I carried out my obs as usual. A worried-looking lady in a pretty headscarf - perhaps his daughter - mentioned in good English that he was a diabetic (type II, non-insulin dependent), so I checked his blood glucose; the meter simply flashed 'LO', which meant his body's sugar level was too low to measure. This was significant and would explain his current state. He had also had a fall earlier in the day, so there was the possibility of a head injury.

The other paramedic's crewmate had arrived, carrying the chair and panting, and we wasted no more time with the patient. He was given oxygen and taken down to the ambulance as quickly as possible. Luckily (and thankfully), we were shown to the lift - it was on the other side of the building. The man was too floppy to carry down stairs safely, so the lift, regardless of the distance we had to run with him to get to it, was a blessing.

Once in the ambulance, I gave him an injection of Glucagon and the other paramedic started running glucose fluids IV. The combination would release stored sugar and boost the blood glucose level immediately. If we had this wrong, there would be no improvement. If we had it right, he would revive quite quickly.

Meanwhile, lots of members of his family had started gathering outside the ambulance. A young man pushed his way to the front and, very politely, said, 'How is my grandfather, please?'

I left the other paramedic working on him and stepped down from the vehicle. Speaking to the young man and the woman in the headscarf, I said, 'His blood sugar was very low, so we're trying to get that up. And we're giving him oxygen. He's in good hands.'

Some of them spoke no English, so the message was quickly relayed around the group and I saw them begin to relax slightly. People want confidence in a crisis; they place their trust in you and you do your best by them. It's a humbling feeling.

Inside, the man was beginning to show signs of improvement. His breathing was still being supported but he was definitely fighting for himself. I re-tested his blood glucose and this time the meter read '1.3', which is very low but an increase on my last result. 'He's getting better,' I shouted to the young man, and a smile of relief passed across his face. Mentally, I began to relax slightly, too.

I travelled with the patient in the ambulance and his glucose level had risen to above 7 by the time he reached hospital. We still didn't know if this was the only cause of his sudden deterioration, but it looked very likely. Somewhere along the line, the man had neglected himself; it's important for type II diabetics to watch what they eat and when they eat it, and any lapse can be serious.

After we handed him over - confident that he was going to be OK now - I couldn't help reflecting on how time-critical this call had been. If the layout of that estate hadn't been so difficult to understand, we would probably have got to the man before he lost consciousness. Conversely, the stupidity of the place's design could have contributed to a delay which cost him his life. Badly put-together housing is another way, less obvious than others, in which the poor and weak have the odds stacked against them.

Unfortunately, the poor are always calling ambulances, sometimes when they don't really need them. The only thing more frustrating than spending precious time trying to find a seriously-ill person on an estate which might have been put together by Salvador Dali is spending precious time trying to find someone who isn't ill at all.

I was working on an ambulance in east London when an emergency call came in for a 22-year-old female with severe DIB. We rushed to the scene and found ourselves staring up at a block of flats which may or may not have been the caller's location. We struggled through a locked gate on every flight of steps (and there were lots of them) until we reached the top floor of the building.

There we found a young woman. She came towards us, shuffling her feet and coughing. She got right up to us before either of us spoke; we were too busy staring at her in disbelief. We knew what was coming.

'Did you call us?' my colleague asked.

'Yes,' the shuffling girl replied, pulling a tatty green cardigan tighter round her shoulders.

'What for? I mean, what's wrong with you?'

'I'm ill, man. I have a terrible cough and a sore throat.'

'So you think you need an ambulance?'

'Well, yeah. I ain't got no car.'

I looked at my colleague and he looked at me. In irritated astonishment. The one thing this call had had going for it was that our severe DIB wasn't going to have to spend long in the ambulance, because this block directly overlooked the local A&E department. The cheek of this woman was amazing: she honestly thought we were going to take her down stairs, into the ambulance and across the road, literally, to the doors of Accident and Emergency.

'You don't need an ambulance, you only have a cold,' said my crewmate.

'Whaa?' said the girl, her face twisting into a mask of aggression. 'You have to take me, it's the law.'

'No we don't, and no it isn't.'

That stumped her for a moment. She coughed a bit, and sniffled. Then she said, 'Well, what are you going to do, then?'

We took her temperature (normal), checked her pulse (normal) and listened to her chest (slightly wheezy).

'If you want to go to hospital,' said my colleague, 'and I don't think you need to but that's by the by, then get a taxi. Or walk.'

We left.

Piling insult upon absurdity, as we walked away she pulled out her mobile phone and called her boyfriend to come and pick her up instead. He lived in the next block, and was waiting at the bottom, engine running, before we even got down.

THE HISTORY OF STRANGERS

I love my job, and I hope that has come across in these pages. Yes, there are frustrations and irritations, and we see some terrible things. It's certainly not the exposure to violence, the drunken idiots, the senseless deaths and the smells and stains associated with bodily fluids. There's just something about the job, something intangible that I can't quite explain, that makes it almost addictive. It gets under your skin.

It's interesting, it can be exciting at times, and it's varied, because you never know what you will be dealing with next. Sometimes, you get to save a child's life while the mother watches. But there is another aspect of the job that draws me to it. People.

If you asked anyone who knows me well enough they will tell you that I don't actually socialise much. I'm not good at the whole getting together in a group thing. To an extent, that's true - I like my privacy and I don't agree with the common viewpoint all the time. I have my own ideas, beliefs and theories for everything in the Universe. I'm not a loner and I have a good circle of friends - I'm just not a party animal and I like to get home after work and relax with my other half and a cat with attitude called Scruffs.

Being a paramedic allows me the honour of walking across a stranger's threshold and into their private lives. I get to see their memories in photographs and hear their tales and experiences first hand.

A lot of the houses I walk into are horrible places in which to live and many of the individuals I have dealt with are not the kind of people I would normally get on with. Of course, there are a few that I don't get on with even as a paramedic, simply because they are bad people to start with, but more often than not I will walk into a home, horrible or not, where I will meet the nicest people you can imagine.

I work hard at my job, and I only really get rewarded when someone says 'Thank you'. We all feel better when a patient or their relative says this - it validates what we are doing and doesn't make the job such a lost cause when we are depressed about how the shift is going.

When I was young, my best friend and I were given the job of mowing the lawn and cutting back the shrubbery of a council house in which a family lived. The single mother was getting the job done for free and it had been arranged by my friend's mum, who was a social worker.

We worked hard all day on that garden; if it wasn't tidied up, the young woman and her kids would be thrown out. It was summer and the heat was relentless, making us sweat and exhausting us by the end of the task.

We went into the woman's house and she sat us down and offered us a cheese sandwich. We hadn't eaten all day, nor had we been offered anything until that point. I heard one of her children complain that she couldn't 'give all their food away'. I asked her what that meant and she told me that the bread and cheese she was offering was all that they had to eat until Monday (it was Saturday) when she could collect her benefit money.

My friend and I declined her offer, but I have never forgotten how generous she was prepared to be in order to thank us. She had no other way of showing her appreciation because she had nothing else to give.

I remind myself of her whenever I walk into a home where the family are clearly disadvantaged. I came from a rough Glasgow town and was brought up on a council estate, so I don't have any airs or graces about it. I do, however, understand that a thank you from someone who has nothing is a valuable thing.

I met an old woman from a block of flats in one of those notorious estates in north London once. She was writing her memoirs down, in longhand, using a biro. She was 80 years old, and we were taking her to hospital because she had fallen over and hit her head. I had a long conversation with her and she told me what she did during the war.

'I used to work in a factory,' she said, 'making the little dials for the instruments on fighter planes and bombers.'

My crewmate and I listened with interest as she continued, pride beaming in her aged face.

'We used to have to paint them with special stuff. It was radioactive paint to make the dials luminous. We had no protection, no mask or anything in those days and I used to get home at night and when I put the light out I could see my footprints glowing on the carpet.'

She chuckled to herself, seeing those footprints all over again in her mind's eye. I would never have got to hear that story - or a million others - if I hadn't been doing this job, and it meant a lot to me because it was her life I was hearing about and she thought it was important enough to share - hence, the memoirs.

People of all cultures invite us into their homes and some of the most well-mannered kids I have encountered have been those belonging to Muslim households. I always make a point of apologising for my footwear when I enter a Muslim home because most of them remove their shoes before crossing the threshold. We don't because there is a health and safety issue about it and it would be highly impractical for us. I believe we are going to be issued with shoe covers to resolve this issue.

Muslims are generally very family-orientated and their religion is part of everything they do; it provides them with the tools to lead a good life. This filters through to their children and what you end up with is a foundation for a good society. I am not writing this because there is a political point to be made, or any

227

other rubbish; I'm highlighting the differences I see in people. I will say this, however; it's a shame more of us don't lead a more family-oriented way of life - for many indigenous British people, their kids seem to be the most dangerous thing running around the streets these days. No wonder other cultures look down on us as sloppy disciplinarians.

Some of my colleagues have been offered food, tea and cold drinks just because it is the way of hospitality in some families. I've been offered the most comfortable chair in the room, for example, when I have been treating someone's son. These little gestures are 'thank yous', and we mustn't forget that.

Many street people have histories that are well worth listening to, and can be especially sad.

I sat in the back of an ambulance with a homeless 45-year-old who had called us because he was cold and hungry. He was desperate and had nowhere else to turn, so he dialled 999 and hoped we would be nice to him.

I bought him something to eat, and I checked his temperature and other obs while he ate. We chatted about how he had found himself on the street. I've been there myself - in my early days in London, when I was a teenager, I had to rough it until I found a job - so I was curious about how he had fallen to this.

He told me that he was an accountant and that his wife had left him with three kids to bring up, which he found difficult to do. He quit his job and tried to exist on Social Security payments, but he lapsed into alcoholism when things got real and he found he couldn't cope. He had struggled like this for years until his children had grown up and left home. By then, he had debts and was drinking every day.

After a while, his home was repossessed and he found himself on the street because the council had no statutory duty to house him. He wandered about until he found a place to sleep, and that was pretty much where he'd been ever since.

'How long have you been on the street?' I asked.

'Nine years,' he said. 'Today's my birthday.'

He knew all he was going to get was another chance to sleep outside, but we took him to hospital in the hope that a diagnosis of 'low temperature' was enough to give him a bed for a few hours.

I never saw that man again.

I see a lot of elderly people and not one of them has given me grief without a good reason - such as Alzheimer's. Generally speaking, they are lovely people and a few of them cling to a single memory because it's the only thing they have left to live for.

We were preparing an 85-year-old lady for transfer to a hospice. This meant she was never going to see her home again. She spoke to us at length about her husband and it was fascinating and poignant.

'I met him early in the war when I was 19,' she told us. 'He was an RAF pilot and I thought he was so brave that I fell in love with him immediately. We got married soon after we met and we bought this house. We had a wonderful couple of years together, but then he got killed in action. He was only 23. I never stopped loving him and I miss him every day. Even now.'

She was holding a photograph of him in his RAF uniform, and she showed it to me with pride and love in her eyes. She was standing with him in the picture, looking young and happy, and I realised that this woman had never entertained the thought of another man in her life. She was still married to the airman in the photograph, but he had died 60 or more years ago. She couldn't have known much about him - he would have been in action a lot of the time - but she had loved him so fiercely that she couldn't let go.

As we took her away from her home, the home she had shared with him, I felt a pang of guilt because - the photo and her thin gold wedding ring aside - we were separating her from her last tangible connection to her husband for the final time. I couldn't find the words for her - nothing appropriate could be said, so I continued as if her story had been a pleasant thing to hear. In fact, it was one for the most emotional insights into another human being's life I had ever been privy to.

Interested people usually ask the same question when they want to know about this job. 'What's the worst thing you've ever had to deal with?' they'll ask. I've yet to meet someone who enquires about my best experience.

So far, working in London has given me experience with the worst of society, the horror of violent death and the sadness of suffering that I am exposed to regularly. It is rare to go home with a happy memory - a call that leaves a smile on my face and dissipates the bad stuff.

Bringing a new life into the world gives me a sense of satisfaction, as does saving someone who would certainly have died had I not intervened, and there are often little comedy moments - irony and paradox in the behaviour of some of my patients. Human mistakes I have made in communication and interpretation have given me and others a little light relief. These things come along unexpectedly and are pleasant interludes, but they aren't the gifts we hope for every time we go on duty.

My best experience has nothing to do with patient care. I was asked to become the Training Supervisor (TS) for a newly trained crew during their last few weeks of the course. They would be on an ambulance dealing with real emergency calls for the first time since leaving the classroom and I was to be with them every step of the way.

The two people I spent that month or so with have since become my friends and we have pleasant memories to share of calls with highs and lows, just like every other crew. What made it special for me was that I was able to watch them develop from nervous, inexperienced individuals to caring, thoughtful technicians with an equal love of the job.

Together, we successfully resuscitated a dying woman in the street, carried drunks to hospital, faced aggression and obstruction and cared for more than a hundred patients in need of help. I felt proud to be doing the job alongside them and sharing whatever knowledge I had to the benefit of their confidence and abilities, from driving at high speed to treating children with amputations.

I think we bonded over a short time and became a crew of three before the end of the training period. They are both now fully qualified EMTs and have saved or helped to save more than a few lives. They reminded me of my limitations and brought me down to earth. Every day or night out with them was a pleasure and something I truly looked forward to.

They did something for me that others have been unable to achieve because of the sheer pressure of the work. They made me laugh.

ALREADY PUBLISHED BY MONDAY BOOKS:

IN FOREIGN FIELDS: TRUE STORIES OF AMAZING BRAVERY FROM IRAQ AND AFGHANISTAN
by Dan Collins (£17.99)

The Iraq War has turned into a quagmire of hatred, violence and death. The bloody Afghanistan conflict is equally savage - a seething cauldron of roadside bombs, ambushes and constant danger. Day after day, our soldiers face implacable and ferocious enemy forces in the searing heat and choking dust of two faraway foreign lands. To make matters worse, many feel the public has turned its back on them.

But the young men and women of our armed forces do not have the luxury of deciding where they fight, and in the deserts and towns of Iraq and Afghanistan a new breed of hero is being born.

Blues and Royals Corporal of Horse Andrew Radford ran 70 metres through a hail of machine gun fire and RPGs to rescue a terribly injured colleague.

Royal Marine Sergeant Matt Tomlinson charged machine gun posts during a river ambush outside Fallujah, and saved the lives of the US Marines he was attached to. Parachute Regiment Lieutenant Hugo Farmer led his men in a desperate, three-hour fire-fight against the Taliban - in the same action for which Corporal Bryan Budd was awarded a posthumous Victoria Cross. This list goes on and on - and now, for the first time, they tell their own stories.

In Foreign Fields features 25 medal winners from Iraq and Afghanistan talking, in their own words, about the actions which led to their awards. Modestly, often reluctantly, they explain what it's like at the very sharp end, in the heat of battle with death staring you in the face. If you support our armed forces, you will want to read this modern classic of war reportage.

"Awe-inspiring untold stories... enthralling" - **The Daily Mail**

IN FOREIGN FIELDS

HEROES OF IRAQ AND AFGHANISTAN
IN THEIR OWN WORDS

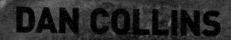

DAN COLLINS

DIARY OF AN ON-CALL GIRL
True Stories From The Front Line
WPC EE Bloggs (£7.99)

If crime is the sickness, WPC Ellie Bloggs is the cure... Well, she is when she's not inside the nick, flirting with male officers, buying doughnuts for the sergeant and hacking her way through a jungle of emails, forms and government targets.

Of course, in amongst the tea-making, gossip and boyfriend trouble, real work sometimes intrudes. Luckily, as a woman, she can multi-task...switching effortlessly between gobby drunks, angry chavs and the merely bonkers. WPC Bloggs is a real-life policewoman, who occasionally arrests some very naughty people. Diary of an On-Call Girl is her hilarious, despairing dispatch from the front line of modern British lunacy.

WARNING: Contains satire, irony and traces of sarcasm.

Based on her hilarious blog about life as a police woman – 'PC Bloggs - a Twenty-First Century Police Officer'

http://pcbloggs.blogspot.com

"Think Belle de Jour meets The Bill... sarky sarges, missing panda cars and wayward MOPS (members of the public)."
- The Guardian

"Part Orwell, part Kafka... and part Trisha."
- The Mail on Sunday

diary of an
ON-CALL GIRL
true stories from
the front line

WPC E.E. BLOGGS

WASTING POLICE TIME...
THE CRAZY WORLD OF THE WAR ON CRIME
PC David Copperfield (£7.99)

PC DAVID COPPERFIELD is an ordinary bobby quietly waging war on crime...when he's not drowning in a sea of paperwork, government initiatives and bogus targets.

Wasting Police Time is his hilarious but shocking picture of life in a modern British town, where teenage yobs terrorise the elderly, drunken couples brawl in front of their children and drug-addicted burglars and muggers roam free.

He reveals how crime is spiralling while millions of pounds in tax is frittered away, and reveals a force which, crushed under mad bureaucracy, is left desperately fiddling the figures.

His book has attracted rave reviews for its dry wit and insight from The Sunday Times, The Guardian, The Observer, The Daily Mail, The Mail on Sunday and The Daily Telegraph;.

'Being a policeman in modern England is not like appearing in an episode of The Sweeney, Inspector Morse or even The Bill, sadly,' says Copperfield. 'No, it's like standing banging your head against a wall, carrying a couple of hundredweight of paperwork on your shoulders, while the house around you burns to the ground.'

"A huge hit... will make you laugh out loud" - **The Daily Mail**
"Very revealing" - **The Daily Telegraph**
"Damning... gallows humour" - **The Sunday Times**
"Graphic, entertaining and sobering" - **The Observer**
"A sensation" - **The Sun**

By PC David Copperfield - as seen on BBC1's *Panorama*

www.coppersblog.blogspot.com

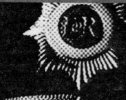

WaStiNG
POLICE
TiMe

the crazy world of the war on crime

PC DAVID COPPERFIELD

IT'S YOUR TIME YOU'RE WASTING
A Teacher's Tales Of Classroom Hell
by Frank Chalk (£7.99)

The blackly humorous diary of a year in teacher's working life. Chalk confiscates porn, booze and trainers, fends off angry parents and worries about the few conscientious pupils he comes across, recording his experiences in a dry and very readable manner. Does for education what PC David Copperfield did for the police.

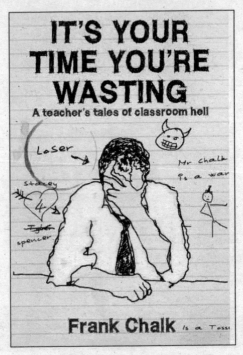

"I recognised many of the situations: the constant cussing between pupils, the back-stabbing staff, colleagues off sick with stress, the aggressive parents, and the ridiculous government bureaucracy and policies." - **The Times**

www.frankchalk.blogspot.com

ROAD TRIP TO HELL:
Tabloid Tales Of Saddam, Iraq And A Bloody War
by Chris Hughes (£7.99)

Tabloid journalist Chris Hughes records his many visits to Iraq pre- and post-war: he finds Saddam's underpants, is carjacked and almost dies and watches US Marines kill unarmed people in a crowd. Visceral and brutal in parts, amusing in others, Hughes is very warm about the Iraqi people and scathing about the US invasion.

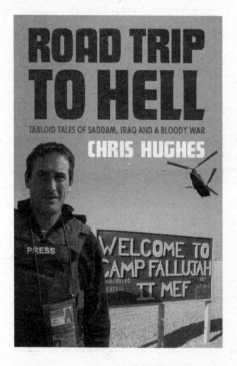

"A brilliant, moving, thought-provoking read" - **The Daily Mirror**

AUSTIN HEALEY is one of English rugby's best-known characters. His extraordinary career has seen him win 50 England caps, star on two British Lions tours and play a leading role in England's most successful club ever – Leicester Tigers – where he won four Premiership titles and two European Championships.

He's rightly regarded as perhaps the most versatile and skilful English player ever and has won fans the world over. But his outspoken nature means he's courted controversy along the way.

In ME AND MY MOUTH, he lays bare the backstage wrangling that bedevilled England's World Cup winners and wrecked those Lions tours – and lifts the lid on the hilarious behind-the-scenes escapades fans rarely get to hear about.

Now with a new career as a BBC TV presenter ahead of him, Austin's sure to stay in the public eye…and this book will ensure he keeps on ruffling feathers.

"More than a mouthful" - **The Daily Telegraph**

"Healey has a natural wit and that comes screaming through"
- The Independent

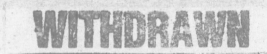